Impact *of* Birthing Practices *on* Breastfeeding

Protecting the Mother and Baby Continuum

Mary Kroeger, BSN, CNM, MPH
with

Linda J. Smith, BSE, FACCE, IBCLC
Bright Future Lactation Resource Centre

JONES AND BARTLETT PUBLISHERS
Sudbury, Massachusetts
BOSTON   TORONTO   LONDON   SINGAPORE

World Headquarters
Jones and Bartlett
  Publishers
40 Tall Pine Drive
Sudbury, MA 01776
978-443-5000
info@jbpub.com
www.jbpub.com

Jones and Bartlett
  Publishers Canada
2406 Nikanna Road
Mississauga, ON L5C 2W6
CANADA

Jones and Bartlett
  Publishers International
Barb House, Barb Mews
London W6 7PA
UK

Cover image © Jan Pana
Copyright © 2004 by Jones and Bartlett Publishers, Inc.

Library of Congress Cataloging-in-Publication Data

Kroeger, Mary.
  Impact of birthing practices on breastfeeding : protecting the mother and baby continuum
/ Mary Kroeger.
     p. ; cm.
  Includes bibliographical references and index.
  ISBN 0-7637-2481-5
     1. Breastfeeding.   2. Childbirth.   3. Childbirth—Social aspects.   I. Title.
     [DNLM: 1. Breast Feeding. 2. Delivery, Obstetric. 3. Maternal Behavior. WS 125 K93i 2003]
  RJ216.K76 2003
  649'.33—dc21

                                                                        2003047492

Acquisitions Editor: Penny M. Glynn
Production Manager: Amy Rose
Associate Production Editor: Renée Sekerak
Editorial Assistant: Amy Sibley
Production Assistant: Tracey Chapman
Associate Marketing Manager: Joy Stark-Vancs
Manufacturing Buyer: Amy Bacus
Composition: Northeast Compositors
Cover Design: Brianna J. Donahue
Printing and Binding: Malloy Incorporated
Cover Printing: Malloy Incorporated

Printed in the United States of America
07 06 05 04 03   10 9 8 7 6 5 4 3 2 1

Dedicated to my mother
Garnett Snedeker Kroeger

CONTENTS

FOREWORD

by Miriam H. Labbok, MD, MPH, FACPM, FABM, IBCLC
Currently Senior Advisor on Infant and Young Child Feeding
and Care, UNICEF New York

Dear Reader:

I am an enthusiast for the mother-child dyad, in recognition of the wonderful interplay of molecules, cells, organ systems, and the interpretations of our lives that make renewal of life seem at once so normal and, yet, so miraculous. As a public health physician, I find myself constantly considering the evolutionary purpose of daily functions: Why do we love to eat sweets and fats? Why do we lust after our mates? Why do we feel safer with our mothers and sisters around us? Why do we feel at peace around a campfire? Why do we fear snakes and spiders? Why do we yawn when others yawn? All of these urges and feelings stem from our evolutionary needs for survival, and our bodies and brains patterns adapted to these needs.

For example, did you know that the vast majority of cultural traditions include support for the mother and child to be isolated from others, and totally supported in terms of household chores and food preparation, for about six weeks postpartum? Why has this phenomenal similarity occurred among diverse and dispersed cultures?

When we see universal cultural practices like this, we again must assume that the origins go beyond a simple matter of communications or personal choice, into the realm of biological and species behavioral evolutionary needs. The probable reason in this case, is that the six weeks corresponds to the time needed for the establishment of lactation and for maternal recovery of uterine tone. Today, however, we expect women to be back at work within days or weeks of delivery, and during that time she is expected to get acquainted with the needs of this child while taking care of many household chores. Is it any surprise that we see innumerable problems with establishing and sustaining lactation?

Midwife, lactation specialist, and international consultant Mary Kroeger has whole-heartedly addressed the conundrum created when contemporary medical and social practices remove us from our biological roots and norms that helped us survive from generation to generation as we evolved as a species.

Evolutionarily speaking, in order to manage to have our large brains, we must deliver our babies when they are quite immature. And this process remains a threat to the survival of mother and baby alike. To overcome the obvious inherent problems, the process of labor must allow the mother's pelvis to relax enough for passage of this large-headed progeny, and then the mother must provide for it until it can fend for itself. We developed internal mechanisms that support this relaxation during labor in spite of the obvious pain and stress, and that create the maternal need to nurture and stay close to the child for many years. These hormonal influences lead one to the other, with those hormones of lactation and attachment the obvious sequel to those of pregnancy, labor, and delivery, and the company of another woman helps us through these times.

It was consideration of this continuum, and the fact that breastfeeding not only nourishes the offspring, but also pleases the mother and delays the next pregnancy, that encouraged me to pursue the development of a method of fertility delay based on breastfeeding. Today, the lactational amenorrhea method (LAM) has undergone clinical trial and is in use in more than forty countries, becoming more and more accepted by mainstream family planning texts. Due to our lifestyles, this method is only reliable for a few months, so it is necessary to include referral to another method for women to achieve the 3-4 years birth spacing that was the norm among our ancestors.

UNICEF recognizes this continuum in the intergeneration lifecycle, and, with the support of the World Alliance for Breastfeeding Advocacy, launched the Golden Bow initiative in 2002. This bow celebrates the mother-child dyad unit, with one loop signifying the mother and the other the child, recognizing in the knot the support of father, family, and society. One ribbon indicates that other foods must be added to breastfeeding after six months, and the other indicates the need for at least three years birth spacing to give time for the mother to recover her nutritional stores, and for the child to be able to begin to care for itself.

The book you are about to experience is both a referenced text and a challenge to our accepted norms. In the enthusiasm to make clear the condition of our health system's active interference with the mother-child dyad, this book occasionally presents historical memories that may differ depending on source, and offers some interpretations of policy decisions that are arguable. But it seems this is done purposefully: Mary Kroeger and her colleague, Linda Smith, constantly challenge us to reconsider what we accept as "normal" healthcare practices and policies.

With recognition and celebration of this natural and necessary continuum of the mother and child, this book offers a stunning argument for respecting the mother-child dyad. The frequent questions put to the reader encourage consideration by the novice, stimulate discussion among those who are informed, and could provoke a healthy, educated argument among the convinced. This is an important book. Whether you agree with the detail, or argue the interpretations, you will have been stimulated to reconsider your medical/nursing/midwifery/lactation management training and will find yourself seeking a better understanding of what is truly the "normal" experience of the human birthing-lactation continuum.

Dear Reader, be ready to re-think what is "normal"...

AUTHOR'S PREFACE

Readers who know midwives know our penchant for telling birth stories, especially stories about difficult births. I am no exception. The story of the "conception, gestation, labor, and birth" in this book goes back more than a decade, to the time when the WHO/UNICEF Baby Friendly Hospital Initiative (BFHI) was launched. BFHI quickly became a global movement, revolutionizing maternity care and providing scientific evidence for best practices in promoting, protecting, and supporting breastfeeding.

Conception - In 1991, I returned to the United States from five years of work overseas with mothers and babies in Central America and Africa. On arrival back to California, where two of my three children had been born, and where I had trained and worked as a maternity nurse and a midwife, I was shocked to see how quickly the nature of birthing had changed during this time. Mothers were increasingly having epidural anesthesia in labor, natural childbirth rooms in many hospitals had closed, and the cesarean section rate had stayed above 23%. I pondered this phenomenon, wondering, what were the forces at work?

Gestation - That year I joined the clinical faculty at Wellstart International in San Diego and worked with the talented and dedicated group of professionals who were providing a model for lactation management education and clinical care that was influencing breastfeeding practices in the USA and globally. As one of the clinicians in Wellstart's "tertiary level" lactation clinic, I saw breastfeeding problems which I had not encountered to any great extent in my developing country work. Many of the babies I saw were from medicated and often obstetrically complicated deliveries. While the babies usually appeared "normal," their breastfeeding was disorganized, at the very least, and sometimes it was seriously dysfunctional. At Wellstart's clinic, we frequently saw mothers who had been discharged home and were in the throws of the typical early postpartum adjustments of sleep deprivation, juggling many new tasks into the former routine, and responding to hormonal changes of the postpartum period. Our intake history form and database included questions about the length of labor, anesthesia used, presence of episiotomy, and method of delivery. Intake information also included how the mother *felt* about her delivery and if she had a sense of pride or failure in her childbirth experience. While there were some mothers and babies seen in the clinic from normal unmedicated vaginal deliveries, they were the minority. Far more mothers had histories of difficulties in labor and had experienced a number of interventions including anesthesia, analgesia, intravenous oxytocin, electronic fetal monitoring, instrumental delivery, and/or cesarean section. It became increasingly clear to me that there likely is a connection between the labor and birth experience and difficulties with breastfeeding.

At this same time, Wellstart International was asked by WHO and UNICEF to help with the development of the BFHI global assessment tools and training courses. During this exciting period, I was included in the strategic discussions about what should be assessed and what should be taught in a BFHI package. As the only obstetric professional on the WSI faculty at that time, I argued strongly for including birthing practices in the BFHI materials. In the end, it was decided that the focus needed to be on the "Ten Steps" as they were, addressing the "baby" and "breastfeeding" constraints. Thus, except for Step Three, which stresses the importance of prenatal education on breastfeeding, the obstetrical component of the mother-baby partnership was omitted.

Early Labor – Determined that this suspected connection might be documented, over the next two years I began collecting research articles whose results shed light on this "missing link" in our breastfeeding support package and set up files on medications, position in labor, support in labor, hydration, and so on. In 1993, I presented a paper at the International Congress of Midwives in Vancouver: *Labor and Delivery Practices: The Eleventh Step to Successful Breastfeeding?* In this paper, I synthesized information gleaned from my critical reading of the literature as well as experience from my then 18 years as a clinician. The paper was well received at the Congress and I submitted it for publication in the *Journal of Nurse Midwifery*. It was not accepted on the grounds that it covered too broad an area of research (which was quite true) and I was invited to re-submit sections of it; for example, limiting discussion to labor medication or cesarean section. In 1995-1996 the *Birth Gazette*, a publication for homebirth- and natural birth-oriented readers, ran parts of the Eleventh Step paper, but it was never published in full. This "early labor" continued over the next few years and by 2000, I had a decade's worth of new publications added to my database.

Hard Labor - In 2001, I was commissioned by the LINKAGES Project, a United States government-funded project for promotion of global breastfeeding, to write a paper reviewing the scientific evidence for linking birthing practices and breastfeeding. This paper, *Birthing Practices and Their Influence on Breastfeeding Success: Review of the Evidence and Recommendations for Developing and Developed Countries* was completed in early 2002. The draft paper was critically reviewed within LINKAGES. While most reviewers thought the paper very interesting and agreed that many links were "suggested" in the literature, LINKAGES ultimately decided that there were still "too many gaps" in solid scientific literature to warrant the paper's publication in their technical paper series.

Transition - It was hard not to be disappointed at this decision, just as with real labor the transition to pushing often comes with discouragement and a feeling of wanting to give up. However, several of the reviewers, particularly those who were in clinical practice providing hands-on help to mothers and babies, urged me to get this paper in print. Special thanks go to Kim Winnard at the LINKAGES Project, to Dr. Audrey Naylor and Ruth Wester at Wellstart International, to Pamela Morrison LLL/I in Zimbabwe, to Dr. Veronica Valdes in Chile, and to Linda J. Smith, at Bright Future Lactation Resource Centre, all of whom encouraged me to push this baby to the light of day.

Birth - It has been a long gestation, a long labor, and an eventful birth. This book is written for obstetricians and pediatricians, anesthesiologists, family practice doctors, midwives, nurses, doulas, childbirth educators, lactation consultants, community-based counselors, researchers, students, mothers, fathers, and families. It attempts to span both developed and developing country settings and thus is also written for global policy setters, program planners, and implementers. It is hoped that this book will spur more perinatal researchers to design studies with breast-feeding as an outcome and others to re-look at existing data that may shed light on this issue. The nature of childbirth and breast-feeding continuum is such that randomized controlled clinical trials may never be able to capture the complete picture. Hopefully more clinicians will come forward to share their observations and case reports. The evidence overwhelmingly suggests that the "best practice" for a maternity care is a holistic, non-invasive model, which is geared to supporting natural processes. Can we afford to postpone mounting an all-out effort (global in scope) to protect mothers, babies, and breastfeeding and to stop the assault on normal, non-invasive childbirth?

Mary Kroeger, BSN, CNM, MPH
Takoma Park, Maryland

PREFACE

by Linda J. Smith

It has been an exhilarating, exhausting, and exciting pleasure to work with Mary Kroeger in creating this book. We have been collecting research, stories, and experiences on the subject for decades, from complementary and slightly different perspectives: Mary as an internationally experienced midwife, and I as a lactation consultant and childbirth educator.

Until fairly recently, breastfeeding care providers assumed that most babies could suck, and that problems were usually maternal issues. However, in my private lactation practice I began encountering a steadily increasing stream of otherwise normal, full-term babies who would start to go to the breast, yet were unable to effectively latch and could not effectively obtain milk. Although weaning to a bottle of formula or pumped milk didn't fix the babies' suck problems, this did accomplish "feeding the baby" which was the mothers' primary, understandable, and legitimate goal. Looking closely at these babies and drawing on my former career as a physical education teacher, I noticed slight to moderate asymmetry in many of them: spinal curvature, asymmetric movements of the limbs, facial asymmetry, and asymmetric tongue movements. Some cried upon flexion, and some had to be held in one specific posture to be able to feed at all.

From April 1990 to April 1993, a chart review of 81 mother-baby pairs who sought lactation consultations for complicated breastfeeding situations related to poor sucking responses yielded the following data: 18 (22%) had oral thrush (Candida) infections; 25 (31%) had asymmetrical posture, overriding cranial sutures, and/or facial asymmetry; 29 (36%) had a short and/or tight lingual frenulum; and 36 (45%) were exposed to epidural anesthesia. After eliminating the tongue-tied babies, 52 remained with impaired sucking response, of which 54% were exposed to epidural anesthesia. The poor sucking was not correctable with improved positioning at breast; most of these babies also had difficulty taking oral fluids by other methods and required extensive therapy.[1]

Parallel to the rise in sucking problems, I noticed that the mothers who elected to use epidural anesthesia/analgesia were not quite as connected to their babies afterward as those who sought unmedicated births. Their commitment and *perseverance* in dealing with breastfeeding problems also seemed weaker or more fragile. However, these were the observations of an experienced educator and breastfeeding care provider, not a scientific study. So I sought physiological explanations and began collecting research related to these observations.

In Chapter 7, I present circumstantial evidence and suggested connections that may begin to make sense of what lactation professionals are encountering in practice: full-term babies who have sucking or other problems related to birth interventions.

---

[1]Bright Future Lactation Resource Centre records provided by author.

AUTHOR'S ACKNOWLEDGEMENTS

Firstly, my deepest thanks go to Linda J. Smith, who was key in convincing me to take the steps to expand my earlier work and research into a full textbook. Linda assisted in so many ways, always available for review, discussion, critique, as well as assistance with research on some topics. As I labored with this book, she served as my "midwife" and offered encouragement when I felt stuck at 8 centimeters with the production. Linda authored Chapter 7, and in it she presents exciting and valuable information on the "forces and physics" of birth and impact on breastfeeding, drawing from her *understanding* of muscles, bones, and nerves, *experience* as a physical education teacher, and years of practice as childbirth educator and lactation consultant.

I want to thank my wonderful husband, Robert Armstrong, who encouraged me, made tea, rubbed my back, and generally was willing to share his wife with a computer for weeks at a time. I wish to thank my three children, Douglas, Adam, and Reva, each of whose births strengthened my trust that childbirth is a natural event. I wish to thank my 8-month old granddaughter, Grace, for her foresight in slipping into my hands and then her mother's arms at home at dawn last summer, when the plan was that she would be born in a maternity facility. Grace's coming this way preserved the mother-baby continuum within my own family.

I want to thank the many colleagues, friends, and former midwifery clients from around the globe who helped in big and small ways to bring this book to its completion. These include:

Ashley Aakensson, Sarah Amin, Gene C. Anderson, Helen Armstrong, Janet Isaacs Ashford, Cherry May Avilez, Jean Baker, Jeannine Parvati Baker, Susan Baker, Tom Bauer, Martin Butcher, Ella and Kara Barcello, Nils Bergman, Hannah Smith Boswell, Lisa Breen, Ann Brownlee, Karin Cadwell, Beverly Chalmers, Mwate Chintu, Maureen Chilila, Annie Clark, Suzanne Colson, Jean Cotterman, Rae Davies, Robbie-Davis Floyd, Eugene Declercq, Susan Fine, Janis Fox-Davis, Marge Freeman, Ann Fulcher, Sister Pat Gage, Ina Mae Gaskin, Henci Goer, Jere Graham, Martha Grodrian, Karen Kerkhoff Gromada, Carole Hagin, Doris Haire, Maggie and Steve Hall, Adrianne L. Harrington, Barbara Heiser, Justus Hofmeyr, Jenna Houston, Deborah Humphreys, Kate M. Jones, Timothy Kachule, Dennis Keating, Sheila Kitzinger, Kip Kozlowski, Bob Kroeger, Miriam Labbok, Minda Lazarov, Nikki Lee, Adik Levin, Ruowei (Rosie) Li, Robin Lim, Banyana Madi, Rebecca Magalhaes, Jean A. Maloni, Margaret Maimbolwa, Susan Mann, Kay Martin, Luann Martin, Dorla McKenzie, Lisa Mecca, Anne Merewood, Eva Middleton, Pamela Morrison, Altrena Mukuria, Maureen Mzumara, Audrey Naylor, Edward R. Newton, Karen L. Newton, Laurie Nommsen-Rivers, Nomajoni Ntombela, Tina Nyirenda, Judith O'Connell, Michel Odent, Ana Parrilla, Jose Gorrin Peralta, Nancy Powers, Edda Pugin, Carol Sakala, Lisa Sandora, Roberta Scaer, Ma Sedta, Kate Sharp, Susan Siew, Penny Simkin, Wendy Slusser, Mary Smith, Meena Sobsamai, Adwoa Steel, Maryanne Stone-Jimenez, Carole Thomason, Marian Tompson, Veronica Valdes, Marsden Wagner, Ruth Wester, Kim Winnard, and Vincenzo Zanardo.

Thanks to all the mothers, grandmothers, and midwives in Cambodia, China, Ghana, Indonesia, Kazakhstan, Malawi, and Zambia who gave verbal permission, through translators, for me to use their photographs for the purpose of teaching and improving maternal and infant health globally.

Finally, thanks to my mother, Garnett S. Kroeger, who always told me I could do anything I put my mind to do.

CHAPTER 1

CHILDBIRTH AND BREASTFEEDING IN A HISTORICAL CONTEXT

"The childbirth practices of a nation [are] the reflections of that nation's beliefs concerning the integrity and dignity of life, and [influence] that nation for good or evil, and ultimately the world itself..."

Dr. Grantly Dick-Read

Homebirth and Institutional Birth

Until early in the twentieth century, women nearly everywhere labored and delivered at home, and breastfeeding was for them a normal part of the reproductive process. In the home environment, a woman would labor and deliver without medical intervention, typically with the support of relatives and/or a familiar, empirically trained birth attendant. In this setting, assuming the labor and birth progressed normally, the mother-baby partnership was protected and breastfeeding was initiated and sustained for several years. Homebirth without the help of a skilled provider had its downside; if there were serious complications for the baby or the mother, the lack of immediate access to appropriate referral facilities, to skilled care providers, and to modern medicines meant that it was not uncommon for newborn, mother, or both to die during or after the birth.

The transition from homebirth to facility-based birth as the norm has occurred at different rates and in different ways from country to country, and from continent to continent. On some continents, Africa for example, more than half of all babies still are born at home. Exploring all these trends is beyond the scope of this book, but because of the global emphasis on breastfeeding promotion, there will be an attempt to compare developed country trends, particularly trends in the United States, with those of the developing world.

By the end of World War II, childbirth in the hospital had become the norm in the United States. The exception to this was the rural, racially segregated South, where lay midwives continued to practice until they were outlawed in the 1970s.[1] These "Grand" midwives, trained mostly by their own mothers and grandmothers, provided pregnancy, homebirth, and postpartum care to the African-American and poor white communities. In the 1970s, state-by-state, authorities decided they were a threat to public health and their licenses were revoked (Figure 1-1).[2] Throughout the 1940s to 1960s, in the United States most women were attended at birth by a physician, with nurses providing the labor care in a scenario much like the one that follows: With the onset of labor, a pregnant woman would be admitted to a maternity hospital and "prepped" by having all pubic hair shaved and frequently she was given an

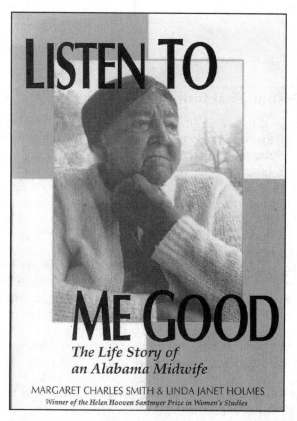

FIGURE 1-1 Margaret Smith practiced as a homebirth midwife in rural Alabama for over 30 years. In *Listen to me Good* she tells her story, with the assistance of Linda J. Holmes.

enema. She would labor alone, usually in bed, and would be allowed nothing to eat or drink. For pain relief, she most likely was offered meperidine injections (commercially known as Demerol or as Pethidine in Europe), or another combination of morphine (a narcotic) and scopolamine (an amnesiac), resulting in a state known as "twilight sleep." For the delivery she might be asked to breathe nitrous oxide or ether, or be given a spinal block of some kind, numbing her from the waist down. Gradually, as research began to link these medicines to labor dysfunction, maternal disorientation and hallucination, and to fetal asphyxia, they were replaced with newer narcotic drugs: alphaprodine (Nisentil), butorphanol (Stadol) and nalbuphine (Nubain). These medicines had the desired pain relief effects but were claimed to be shorter acting and safer.

At the time of delivery, a mother would deliver in the lithotomy position, flat on her back with legs in stirrups and perhaps with her hands in restraints (Figure 1.2). It was routine for an episiotomy to be performed and for forceps to be used because the mother might not be able to bear down herself. Her baby, delivered by the doctor, would have its mouth suctioned, be held upside down and "spanked" on the buttocks to stimulate crying, and then be handed to the nurse. The nurse would move the baby to a separate heated crib and would begin admission procedures which would include silver nitrate eye drops (which burn), umbilical cord care, foot print-ing, weighing, measuring, Vitamin K injection, and sometimes other lab tests that required puncturing the newborn's heel to obtain blood. The baby would be bathed from head to toe, removing the naturally protective vernix (a white, waxy lubricant on the skin now known to be anti-infective), and then diapered and dressed.

The mother was usually not allowed to hold the baby until she was transferred to the postpartum ward; it was common for a mother not to see her baby until hours after the delivery. In the newborn nursery, the baby would undergo "observation" by the staff. Commonly the baby was given a "test feed " of sterile water to ensure that no congenital tracheoesophageal fistula existed (a rare hole in the baby's throat area that could lead to choking). Even if the mother planned to breastfeed, depending on the time of day or night, glucose water or formula was given in the nurs-ery as a first feed, while the mother "rested."

This model of obstetrical care remained the norm in the United States for several decades, and was exported to medical training institutions and hospitals throughout the developing world. In contrast, in Europe, particularly in the Netherlands, Eng-land, and the Scandinavian countries, midwives were more likely to be the attendants of normal birth. In these settings, the use of medical techniques, including routine episiotomy and drugs in labor, were less common.

Natural Childbirth Movement in the West

By the late 1950s, a small minority of mothers began questioning their childbirth care. The "natural childbirth movement" should probably acknowledge Dr. Grantly Dick-Read as its unofficial founder. Dick-Read, a British obstetrician who had attended many births at home in England in the 1930s and 1940s, recognized that in the home environment women birthed more naturally, apparently free of fear and the need for pain medication. He compared his homebirth patients to those he attended in the hospital and concluded that much of the fear and pain of childbirth was reinforced by the hospital environment and hospital birth attendants who isolated the mother in labor and offered chloroform or other labor narcotics for the pain rather than touch, support, and encouragement. In 1944, he published *Childbirth Without Fear: The Principles and Practice of Natural Childbirth.*[4] This book, read

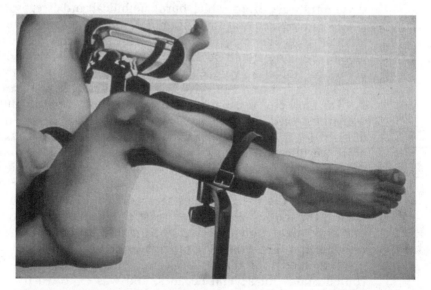

FIGURE 1-2   The lithotomy position for delivery. *Source:* Ashford JI.1986. Booklet and Slide set: *Mothers and Midwives: A History of Traditional Childbirth.* Self Published., Out of Print.[3]

by American women as well as by women in England and the rest of Europe, set the stage for others who had begun questioning obstetric practices in American hospitals. The book not only describes the physiologic basis of how fear can interfere with labor and increase pain and anxiety, it also gives relaxation techniques and exercises. Dick-Read stresses the need for continual comfort and support during labor, an idea several decades ahead of the studies that show conclusively that continuous labor support reduces need for many labor interventions, including pain medication (See Chapter 3).

The revised second edition of Dick-Read's book was published in 1959. That same year, Marjorie Karmel, an American woman who had sought and found an alternative to medicalized childbirth, published *Thank You, Dr. Lamaze*. This book, which describes Karmel's first delivery in Paris, France, and her second in New York City, set the stage for what was one of the first childbirth preparation movements in the United States. The "Lamaze method" of prepared childbirth is based on the Pavlovian principles of conditioned reflexes.[5] The method argues that if women are "conditioned" to expect pain with uterine contractions, they will indeed experience pain, but if they are deconditioned through education and support and relaxation in labor, the pain can be averted. Using the technique of psychoprophylaxis, the method teaches that, with practice, a laboring mother can use prelearned breathing and relaxation techniques during contractions to keep the pain under control. As her labor becomes stronger, she changes the breathing to a different and more complex pattern to accommodate the increasing intensity and uses an additional breathing pattern for pushing. Integral to the method is a supportive labor coach who assists in reminding the mother to breathe, to rest between contractions, and to change breathing patterns when it seems necessary.

In the introduction to the second edition of *Thank You, Dr. Lamaze* (1981), Elisabeth Bing, herself a pioneer in childbirth education, writes that Karmel's book and courageous personal testimonials to the effectiveness of the Lamaze method ultimately helped American women and their partners to "become the proselytizers of an entirely new approach to childbirth." Bing points out that just months after the publication of the first edition in 1959, the American Society of Psychoprophylaxis in Obstetrics (ASPO) was founded. In 1960, the International Childbirth Education Association (ICEA) was established as the first international childbirth organization. Both shared the mutual aims of furthering natural, family-centered maternity care.

La Leche League International

In its early years, La Leche League International (LLL/I) played a significant role in the United States in making links between natural childbirth and breastfeeding. In 1957, seven women with families in suburban Chicago, Illinois founded LLL/I, an organization whose main mission was and still is to provide information and support through personal help to mothers and families to enable successful breastfeeding (Figure 1-3). Among the seven LLL/I founders was Mary White, who was married to doctor Gregory White, a doctor trained in family medicine and obstetrics. Dr. White's practice, somewhat unique in his suburban neighborhood of Franklin Park, promoted the practices of unmedicated childbirth and breastfeeding; he also attended births at home.[6] In 1955, Marian Tompson, who later became the first president of LLL, looked for a doctor who could provide a homebirth for her fourth baby. Her first three children had been born in a natural manner in a hospital without drugs, but her husband had been excluded from the deliveries. Dr. White agreed to attend her birth at home, and with her husband's help she delivered and breastfed her fourth child with ease. She went on to deliver all of her last four babies with Dr. White. Six of the seven LLL Founders had homebirths with Dr. White for their subsequent babies. In fact, eight of the White's eleven children were home born and all were breastfed.[7]

The LLL/I mother-to-mother support group model, which has become their hallmark, includes four basic mothers meetings, with a different topic for each discussion. In 1956 these topics were: 1) Advantages of Breastfeeding, 2) Overcoming Difficulties, 3) The Arrival of the Baby, and 4) Nutrition and Weaning. The third meeting included a discussion of the natural approach to birth and the importance of early contact with the baby and early breastfeeding.[8] This information was highlighted because most mothers coming to these meetings in the early years had experienced medicated births and had no idea that this might have a deleterious effect on breastfeeding. In 1957, LLL/I sponsored Dr. Grantly Dick-Read to speak in Franklin Park. There were no funds to pay his (then hefty) $750 speaker's fee, but they rented a school auditorium that held 1250 people and took a chance that charging one dollar per person would partly cover the costs. The auditorium was filled to capacity and many were turned away due to the advertising the founders had done and the eagerness of area families to learn more about the advantages of natural birth and breastfeeding. The success of the evening left them with a growing membership and a net profit of $350.

Early LLL literature made direct links between birth and early breastfeeding. The loose-leaf booklet that predates the bound and published second edition of *The Womanly Art of Breastfeeding* includes the section "Does the Type of Delivery Affect Breastfeeding," which reads:

> Hand in hand with breastfeeding goes a natural delivery. Just as a woman takes pride in carrying her child and later in feeding him herself, so too should she take pride in giving birth to him. Childbirth is a woman's natural function. It is hard work, but a job well worth doing. We who have been allowed to do the job ourselves can only say that the joy in being awake to hear our baby's first cry is the crowning moment of achievement. Our feelings towards our baby make us want to hold him close and put him to the breast at once. This, needless to say, encourages the milk to come in sooner and with both baby and mother feeling well and strong the nursing is bound to be more successful.[9]

The second edition of *Womanly Art of Breastfeeding,* bound and first published in 1963,[10] has clear guidance to mothers on the advantages of a normal, "natural" childbirth both for the mother and the newborn, and for breastfeeding. Expectant mothers are

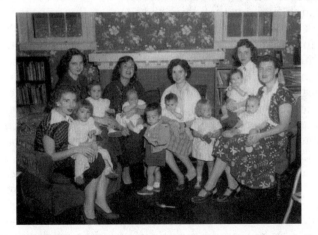

FIGURE 1-3   La Leche League Founders with their small children: Left to right - Mary Ann Cahill, Betty Wagner Spandikow, Mary Ann Kerwin, Mary White, Marian Tompson and Edwina Froehlich. Co-Founder Viola Lennon is not included. *Photo courtesy of LLL/I.*

encouraged to seek out childbirth education with ASPO (Lamaze) and the ICEA. A reference list is provided which includes Dick-Read and other early natural childbirth proponents. The book promotes "alert participation" in the birth, the supportive presence of one's husband, and the immediate holding and breastfeeding of the baby. These recommendations predate by almost three decades the "early initiation" recommendation of the Baby Friendly Hospital Initiative, launched by UNICEF and the World Health Organization in 1991 (See pages 19–20 for BFHI).

In 1964, LLL/I held its first convention in downtown Chicago. Estimates were that 150 mothers would attend, but in fact 450 mothers attended along with 100 infants. Among the featured speakers were several who addressed issues of childbirth. These included the behavioral scientist Niles Newton, and two doctors who practiced obstetrics, Dr. Gregory White and Dr. Robert Bradley. Bradley pioneered the "husband coached childbirth" model. Other speakers included a local nurse and childbirth educator, Margaret Gamper, and the then president of ICEA, Helen Wessel. This first conference saw that including birth issues was a priority.

As the LLL/I membership grew, the need arose for additional literature geared not only to mothers, but also to health providers. In their Information Sheet Series, Info Sheet Number 20 "Together, and Nursing, from Birth" addressed birth and breastfeeding. These info sheets drew on current scientific research and, as early as 1972, cited research findings that described the negative impact of labor pain medicines on early breastfeeding. Research from Russia done in 1955 documented that the sucking reflex is at its height 20–30 minutes after birth[11] arguing for immediate mother-baby contact after birth. The 1978 revised version of Info Sheet No. 20 presents 28 scholarly references on the evidence for noninterference in the mother and newborn continuum and for early and extended contact between mother and her newborn.[12] LLL/I led the way in both the popular and scientific communities in advocating natural birth, breastfeeding, and keeping mother and baby together.

Since 1957, the LLL/I has accredited over 30,000 Leaders, and currently there are over 6400 who are active. There are 2550 mother-to-mother support groups in 65 countries.[13] Their "Position and Philosophy Statement" still includes as one of the ten key points the "alert and active participation by the mother in childbirth [as] a help in getting breastfeeding off to a good start."[14] However, LLL/I has also evolved with the times on the question of childbirth links to breastfeeding. The fifth edition of *The Womanly Art of Breastfeeding,* like the second edition 30 years earlier, has a chapter about planning for baby, now called "Plans are Under-

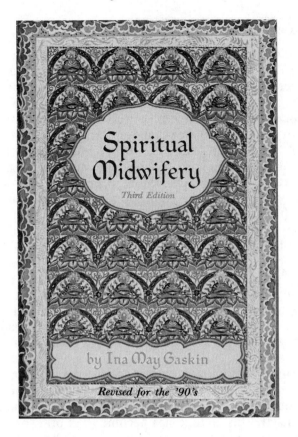

FIGURE 1-4　*Spiritual Midwifery* by Ina May Gaskin influenced the resurgence of midwifery and homebirth in the United States and around the world.

way."[15] In this updated chapter the option of a "trained midwife" as birth attendant and a "birth center" setting are described. One couple's positive experience with a birth center is presented, emphasizing their appreciation for the quiet, intimacy, and lack of medical interference. One section describes the quadrupling of the cesarean section rate in the United States between 1970 and 1987, and references are given for cesarean prevention options in the back of this edition. However, not mentioned at all are some of the iatrogenic reasons for this rising C-section rate. Nor is there a section that describes clearly the disadvantages and side effects of invasive medical interventions and labor medications, including epidural anesthesia, on the baby and breastfeeding.

The Natural Childbirth Movement Grows

The natural childbirth movement flourished in the United States during the 1970s and early 1980s. Popular books, aimed at the consumer, were published and read by a growing constituency of families who wanted more control over their childbirth and breastfeeding experiences (see Box 1-1). Hospitals began to build "natural birth rooms," and free-standing birth centers began to spring up. A small, significant group of childbearing families sought birth at home, and midwives began to make their entrance as maternity care providers. Licensed nurse midwives began practicing in a few urban hospitals and in underserved communities. Direct-entry (unlicensed) midwives began to attend homebirths, often with only a medical text from a local library as a guide. Ina May Gaskin's book, *Spiritual Midwifery* published in 1975, served as the handbook for many of these self-appointed homebirth (Figure 1-4).[16] A sad historic irony is that while a small, but significant group of largely white, middle-class families were reawakening to the advantages of natural childbirth and homebirth, the last of the community-based midwives, who had provided this very service in the states of the deep South, were being legally eliminated.[2]

One consumer battle that was hard fought and won was gaining permission for continuous support in labor by partners and other family members, first in the labor room and eventually for the delivery itself. This change has become the norm for care in U.S. hospitals. Gradually, even partners of mothers who had cesarean sections were allowed to don "scrub suits" and watch their newborns be surgically delivered.

Box 1-1

Selected books on childbirth and newborns published between 1970 and 1990 that were significant in the rise of the natural childbirth and homebirth movements in the United States and elsewhere. The first editions of some are now considered classics.

1972   *The Cultural Warping of Childbirth,* by Doris Haire

1972   *The Experience of Childbirth* (U.S. publication), by Sheila Kitzinger

1972   *Birth Book,* by Raven Lang

1973	*Our Bodies, Ourselves: A Book by and for Women,* by Boston Women's Health Collective
1973	*Witches, Midwives, and Nurses: A History of Women Healers,* by Barbara Ehrenreich and Deidre English
1975	*Immaculate Deception: A New Look at Women and Childbirth in America,* by Suzanne Arms
1975	*Birth Without Violence,* by Frederick Leboyer
1977	*Spiritual Midwifery,* by Ina May Gaskin (Figure 1.4)
1979	*Special Delivery: The Complete Guide to Informed Birth,* by Rahima Baldwin
1982	*In Labor: Women and Power in the Birthplace,* by Barbara Katz Rothman
1983	*Bonding the Beginnings of Parent-Infant Attachment,* by Marshall Klaus and John Kennell
1983	*Silent Knife: Cesarean Prevention and Vaginal Birth after Cesarean (VBAC),* by Nancy Wainer Cohen
1984	*A Good Birth, A Safe Birth,* by Diana Korte and Roberta Scaer
1984	*Pregnancy, Childbirth and the Newborn: The Complete Guide,* by Penny Simkin, Janet Whalley, and Ann Keppler
1984	*Birth Reborn,* by Michel Odent
1985	*The Amazing Newborn,* by Marshall Klaus and Phyllis Klaus
1988	*Babies Remember Birth and Other Extraordinary Scientific Discoveries about the Mind and the Personality of Your Newborn,* by David Chamberlain

Another change mothers battled for, and eventually were granted, was being allowed to hold and breastfeed their newborns immediately after birth. Hospitals were very used to the routine of separating newborns from their mothers right after delivery for observation and a myriad of routine procedures. The benefits of this early mother-baby contact, popularly called *bonding,* eventually gained scientific credibility, thanks to the work of Marshall Klaus and John Kennell.[17]

In 1976, a large health maintenance organization in Oakland, California, instituted a special childbirth program called "Shared Beginnings" for families seeking a nonmedicalized childbirth.[18] In this program pregnant women arranged to pay privately for a special maternity nurse to be present for support in advanced labor and delivery, and to assist with the recovery of mother and baby together, thus facilitating early bonding and breastfeeding. Partners were allowed to be part of this process if they could show documentation of attendance at a childbirth preparation class. The mother, partner, and newborn were "allowed" to remain together for the first four hours after delivery in a special recovery room where the Shared Beginnings nurse monitored vital signs, and postpartum bleeding, and helped with initiation of breastfeeding. It was while working as a Shared Beginnings nurse that the author first noticed the marked differences between newborns of mothers who had received medication compared to those who had not. Newborns from unmedicated labors stabilized their temperature, respirations, and heart rate more quickly, and breastfeeding initiation was far quicker and more successful (Figure 1-5).

During this natural childbirth era, there was a simultaneous resurgence in breastfeeding in the United States, with the percentage of women who ever breastfed rising from an all-time low of 22% in 1972 to a peak of 56.3% in 1987 (Figure 1-6). It is inter-

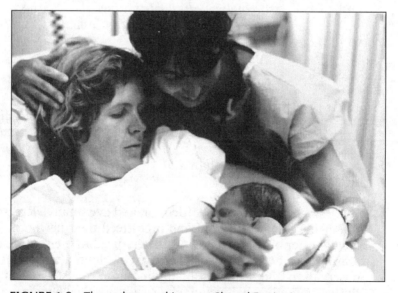

FIGURE 1-5   The author, working as a Shared Beginnings nurse, recovers mother and newborn and assists with first breastfeed at Kaiser Permanente, Oakland 1980. *Photo by Dennis Keating.*

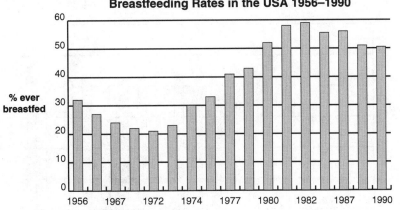

Data Source: *Nat'l Survey of Family Health (1956–87) and Ross Laboratories (1988–90)[19]*

FIGURE 1-6 Breastfeeding rates in the United States began to climb in the early 1970s at the same time that the natural childbirth movement began to get national attention through consumer movements and popular books. (See Box 1-1.)

esting to compare this trend in breastfeeding with the dates of publication of the childbirth books listed in Box 1-1. Events in the late 1980s began to reverse the trend in natural childbirth and, not surprisingly, breastfeeding rates started to drop again.

Many books, including later editions of the natural childbirth "classics," document the continued battle between an increasingly medically invasive model and a natural, family-centered childbirth model. Authors such as anthropologist Robbie Davis-Floyd,[20] childbirth activist Nancy Wainer Cohen,[21] journalist Jessica Mitford,[22] and sociologist Robbie Pfeufer Kahn,[23] all wrote about the political, financial, and cultural forces at play in the defining standards for a normal birth in the early 1990s. By the mid-1990s, the trend in the United States towards natural birth began to reverse as more and more women accepted routine IV's, electronic fetal monitoring, and epidural anesthesia as a "safe way" to reduce the pain of labor. The rise in medical malpractice insurance premiums gave doctors and hospitals the justification for insisting on electronic fetal monitoring to ensure a continuous paper documentation of labor events and the Cesarean section rate rose sharply (Figure 1-7). During this time, hospitals actually closed their alternative birthing rooms and set up LDR rooms (labor, delivery, recovery), which had the advantage of keeping women in one place for the entire labor and delivery. These newer rooms, often furnished with tasteful wood furniture

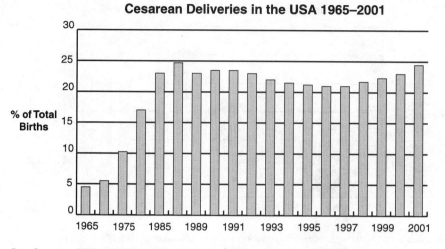

Data Sources: CDC 1995 (1965–88), NCHS Hospital Discharge Surveys (1989–94), and National Vital Statistics Reports (1995–2001)

FIGURE 1-7 Cesarean section rates rose sharply, climbing from 4.5% of all births in 1965 to 16.5% in 1980 and to 24.7% in 1988. The rates declined slightly in the early 1990s as more women sought vaginal birth after a primary C-section (VBAC), but the rates are climbing again, and in 2001 the rate was back to 24.45% of all births.[24]

and soothing artwork, had a homey atmosphere, but also had all the medical technology (the electronic monitors, the epidural trays, and the newborn resuscitation table) stored in bedside closets and cupboards in case they were needed.

Breastfeeding Success Separate from the Birth Continuum?

Breastfeeding rates in the United States, having dropped back some in 1989 and the early 1990s, have continued to stay at the 54-59% rate of mothers who have "ever" breastfed. There are several possible reasons for the gradual rise in breastfeeding rates in recent years. In 1989, the WIC Program (Women, Infants, and Children), a U.S. Department of Agriculture program that supports supplemental nutrition for low-income children, infants, and pregnant and lactating women, initiated a major program shift.[25] WIC, known to be the single largest purchaser of breast milk substitutes in the United States, was accused by breastfeeding advocates of influencing its program members to formula feed through the WIC vouchers, which enable purchase of free formula. In 1989, WIC initiated a campaign to strengthen promotion of breastfeeding among WIC clients and authorized the use of their nutrition services and funds to support a variety of breastfeeding activities. Breastfeeding mothers who were WIC clients became eligible for extra nutrition supplements, and breastfeeding aids, such as pumps, began to be covered by the WIC program. With these program changes, more WIC clients chose to breastfeed.

The American Academy of Pediatrics, having gone on record in 1977 in strong support of breastfeeding, issued a stronger policy statement in 1997, *Breastfeeding and the Use of Human Milk*. The conclusion of this statement calls on pediatrics as a profession to promote and support breastfeeding:

> Although economic, cultural, and political pressures often confound decisions about infant feeding, the AAP firmly adheres to the position that breastfeeding ensures the best possible health as well as the best developmental and psychosocial outcomes for the infant. Enthusiastic support and involvement of pediatricians in the promotion and practice of breastfeeding is essential to the achievement of optimal infant and child health, growth, and development.[26]

In 1985, lactation consultants became part of the health care team. The same year, the International Lactation Consultant Association held its founding meeting in Washington, DC, and began publication of the *Journal of Human Lactation,* the first peer-reviewed professional journal dedicated solely to human lactation. Although breastfeeding care is part of the scope of practice of physicians, midwives, nurses, dietitians, and other health care providers, breastfeeding care is the entire scope of practice of lactation consultants. The International Board of Lactation Consultant Examiners (IBLCE) has administered its international certifying exam for professional lactation consultants in 11 languages (Arabic, Dutch, English, French, German, Icelandic, Italian, Japanese, Korean, Portuguese, and Spanish) in more than 40 countries across all major continents. As of early 2003, over 12,000 IBLCE certified consultants provide direct clinical support to breastfeeding women in a diverse range of clinical settings, including hospitals, clinics, physician's offices, private practices, and educational settings.[27]

The United States launch of the Baby Friendly Hospital Initiative in 1992 necessitated a federally funded "feasibility study" before implementation became formalized in 1997. By 2000, 68.4% of mothers in the United States had ever breastfed[28] and 31.4% of all mothers were still breastfeeding at three months, a dramatic increase from the 5.4% breastfeeding at three months in 1972. The results of a survey of 1583 women in the United States who had given birth within the last two years conducted by the Maternity Center Association with Harris Interactive showed 59% of woman exclusively breastfeeding at one week after birth and another 19% breast and formula feeding.[29] An impressive 78% of women surveyed were at least partially breastfeeding at one week postpartum.

Is the premise that there is a positive impact of natural birthing on breastfeeding rates no longer valid? Or are there medical, scientific, and consumer movements that essentially support the importance of breastfeeding for infant health, while simultaneously accepting a new definition of "natural and normal childbirth" in the context of maternal health? The Maternity Center Association survey suggests that it is "normal" for one quarter of all American women to deliver by cesarean section, for 53% of all labors to require augmention with oxytocin (pitocin), and for epidural anesthesia to be administered in 63% of all births, 59% of which were vaginal deliveries. Sixty seven percent of mothers surveyed intended to breastfeed their babies. At one week postpartum, 59% reported exclusive breastfeeding. Of the mothers who intended to "fully" breastfeed, 80% reported that they were given or offered free formula samples and nearly half were given formula for supplementation in the hospital. Chapter 12 will present a more detailed discussion of this survey.

A lactation consultant in New York City recently reflected (in an Internet chat room) on the lack of basic information her clients have on the physiology of birth and how much this has changed from her own childbirth experiences 10 and 20 years ago (see Box 1-2).

Box 1-2 Natural Childbirth "Dinosaurs'"?

From Kate Sharp, IBCLC Via the Lactnet

Sent: Tuesday, November 05, 2002 5:54 PM

Subject: Birthing Question

I gave birth 20 years ago at a freestanding birth center with a midwife. The practice was to put the baby to breast "to deliver the placenta." Same thing occurred 10 years ago at home with my son. I work as a private practice lactation consultant with almost all hospital births, and across the board, the mothers have never heard of breastfeeding right away "to deliver the placenta;" they almost all have pitocin [oxytocin] during the labor and virtually all have the IV in for the placenta delivery, with an extra dose of pitocin. Often they really don't know what's in the IV; sometimes the dad knows. I've learned; listen to the dad, the mom doesn't know the details.

There's something really wrong here. I feel very badly about the changes in deliveries and I have a lot of trouble remaining cool, calm, and professional. What will our daughters and daughters-in-law believe, or what will they be told? There was a front-page story in the *New York Times* a while ago about a shortage of pitocin in area hospitals. Oxytocin is produced in women's bodies and we've allowed it to be appropriated by pharmaceutical companies. Of course, if there is bleeding you would use drugs, but what's wrong with nature's plan? So economical, baby feeds, mother moves to the completion of her birth. So beautiful, really, and replaced with a semiconscious mother on an IV that she doesn't control the contents of. Sorry to vent, but I know there are other natural childbirth dinosaurs on the list. Maybe even some young women who know how a natural birth works?[30]

Returning to La Leche League for perspective, it seems this pioneering organization has witnessed the changes described in this chapter. In an interview with one of the more senior staff at LLL/I headquarters, it was learned that three young staff and two close relatives of staff had babies in 2002. Of these, four of the five had cesarean sections and one had a vaginal birth with epidural. Four of the five are breastfeeding.[31] The older LLL/I staff have discussed with concern how this small sampling within their organization may be reflective of the larger picture of birth in the United States today. They conclude that no matter how well prepared a young woman is through LLL/I publications and programs and constant contact with senior staff, she is nonetheless subject to all the routine interventions in childbirth that currently are the norm. She is exposed to what is considered "normal" through the media, maternity care providers, and the expectant mothers' own peers. Younger childbearing mothers are prey to the climate of childbirth as it currently exists in the United States, a climate that fortunately *does* support breastfeeding, but unfortunately *does not* examine the role that childbirth events may play in the breastfeeding experience. One LLL/I Leader and an International Board Certified Lactation Consultant (IBCLC) of many years asks, "Why has a whole new health profession of lactation consultants evolved, when 25 years ago having a neighbor, a mother, or a League Leader in the neighborhood was usually enough to get breastfeeding off to the right start? Are we lactation consultants in business in this country because we are fixing the mess that birth is creating?"[32]

Global Perspective on Birth, Breastfeeding, and Maternal and Infant Survival

Turning from the United States' situation to look across the globe, childbirth in the home is still the norm in most developing and resource-poor countries, in very traditional societies, and in a few industrialized countries, most notably the Netherlands. However, there is an international trend toward discouraging homebirths and institutionalizing the labor and delivery process, even for uncomplicated pregnancies. Seemingly sound reasons are given for this move to the hospital, based on U.S. statistics. In the United States, between 1938 and 1948 there was a shift to hospital birth, with a drop from 45% of all births in the home down to 10%. During that same decade, there was a concomitant drop in maternal mortality of 71% in the United States, a dramatic figure indeed.[33] Infant mortality dropped at a similarly impressive rate.

The situation in developing countries is not so positive. Over the last three decades, international health promotion organizations, including the World Health Organization (WHO) and the United Nations Children's Fund (UNICEF), developed key strategies to decrease infant and child mortality and morbidity worldwide. An early strategic package known as GOBI was actively promoted in the 1980s. and included (G) growth monitoring through routine weighing of infants, (O) oral rehydration therapy (ORT) for diarrhea, (B) breastfeeding promotion, and (I) immunization for prevention of childhood diseases. Although the Expanded Program for Immunization (EPI) produced dramatic increases in immunization coverage worldwide and oral rehydration salts became available in the most remote villages in the world, it was found that breastfeeding rates, particularly in urban areas, were starting to decline.

The Baby Friendly Hospital Initiative

In 1989, UNICEF and WHO issued their joint statement *Protecting, Promoting, and Supporting Breastfeeding: The Special Role of Maternity Services*[34] in which maternity hospitals were targeted for strengthening breastfeeding in the prenatal and early postnatal periods. The rationale for targeting maternity facilities, while recognizing that many births still occur at home, was that if doctors and nurses in the formal health sector established breastfeeding policies and improved practices based on sound evidence, this would ripple out to the community. The joint statement recommended ten principles, applicable in any setting, which came to be known internationally as the "Ten Steps to Successful Breastfeeding" (see Box 1-3).

BOX 1-3   Ten Steps to Successful Breastfeeding (UNICEF, WHO, 1989)

Every facility providing maternity services and care for newborn infants should:

1. Have a written breastfeeding policy that is routinely communicated to all health care staff.
2. Train all health care staff in skills necessary to implement this policy.
3. Inform all pregnant women about the benefits and management of breastfeeding.
4. Help mothers initiate breastfeeding within a half-hour of birth.
5. Show mothers how to breastfeed, and how to maintain lactation, even if they should be separated from their infants.
6. Give newborn infants no food or drink other than breast milk, unless medically indicated.
7. Practice rooming-in—allow mothers and infants to remain together—24 hours a day.
8. Encourage breastfeeding on demand.
9. Give no artificial teats or pacifiers (also called dummies or soothers) to breastfeeding infants.
10. Foster the establishment of breastfeeding support groups and refer mothers to them on discharge from the hospital or clinic.

Soon after this, in 1991, WHO and UNICEF launched the Baby Friendly Hospital Initiative (BFHI) putting forth these "Ten Steps" as international best practices. Global assessment criteria were developed and field-tested in 12 countries. Following this, a major effort by UNICEF field offices led to training health providers in the skills needed to provide optimal breastfeeding care in maternity settings. Among the priority facilities targeted in the early years of BFHI were large government, university, and teaching hospitals, with the intention to influence the academic health sector and thus assist in influencing practice, education, and policy at the country level.

The joint statement document also contains a substantial discussion of the importance of maternal nutrition and health during pregnancy and the impact of labor and delivery management, noting that, "a woman's experience during labour and delivery affects her motivation towards breast-feeding and the ease with which she initiates it."[34] Unfortunately, the BFHI largely omitted any wording or emphasis on maternal health or on labor and delivery, and the focus remained on infant care and breastfeeding. The "Ten Steps" included Step 3, which addresses health education in pregnancy, and Step 4, which addresses early initiation of breastfeeding, but there is no assessment of what occurs during birth. An initiative that could have been the Mother-Baby Friendly Hospital Initiative decidedly left the mother out.

More than a decade has passed since the launch of BFHI, and as of 2002 over 18,000 hospitals and maternity units in 136 countries have been assessed and designated as "baby friendly" according to global BFHI standards.[35] Significant changes in clinical practice worldwide have occurred in the handling of newborns at birth, in early initiation of breastfeeding, in encouraging minimal or no separation of newborns from mothers, and in longer periods of exclusive breastfeeding. However, the same emphasis on protection and support for the mother's health, her emotional integrity, her sense of empowerment, and her participation in decisions about her care, especially during the labor and delivery process, still falls short around the world.

Safe Motherhood Initiative

During the same time frame, the Safe Motherhood Initiative (SMI), launched in 1987 at the International Nairobi Conference on Women, embraced a global commitment to reduce the continued unacceptably high rates of maternal mortality and morbidity in many developing countries. Several years later, the WHO began promoting their "Mother Baby Package," which reemphasizes the key components of the SMI, building on the platforms of equity for women, primary health care, and basic maternity care. From these spring the four pillars of Safe Motherhood: family planning (FP); antenatal care (ANC); clean, safe delivery; and essential obstetric care (EOC).[36]

The pillar of "clean, safe delivery" emphasizes clean and atraumatic delivery with early detection and management of complications at the health center or hospital. In addition, the importance of promotion and support of breastfeeding and management of breastfeeding complications was included in the package. However, not included was a "mother-friendly" pillar, emphasizing privacy and respectful care, encouraging the presence of a supportive relative, and recommending freedom for the mother to move about and choose her own birth position. Nor was there an emphasis on women taking an active role in determining their own priorities and choices for their care. The Safe Motherhood Initiative could be strengthened with a pillar that recognizes

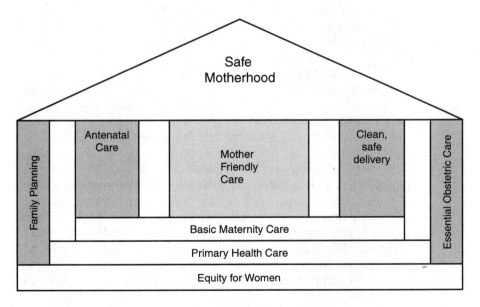

FIGURE 1-8   The four pillars of safe motherhood (WHO,1994). "Mother Friendly" pillar added by author.

that women with risk factors will more likely seek care if they can be assured that care will help them be *safe* (Figure 1-8).

Moving Birth from Home to Facility

At first glance it seems logical that global maternal and child health policy makers would advocate a shift to hospital birth for mothers in the developing world, similar to the shift that occurred in the United States (where maternal mortality rates remain unacceptably high). The "Mother-Baby Package" recommends that birth occur in a health care facility or at least with a formally trained provider and identifies the midwife as the most appropriate and cost-effective type of health provider to be assigned to normal pregnancy, labor, and delivery care. The international definition of a midwife requires that she be trained by an educational program, "recognized by the government that licenses her."[37] Yet, even as the call to move birth to a facility is made, many countries still face a critical shortage of doctors, midwives, and other trained health staff to attend births in referral centers. Those community-based facilities that exist are often distant from remote communities and are inadequately equipped and staffed.

The WHO definition of a trained midwife does not include the preponderance of traditional midwives around the world who have learned childbirth and newborn care from their own mothers and grandmothers or from their own practical experience. This omission creates a program gap since WHO estimates that 53% of all deliveries in the developing world still occur with an untrained birth attendant, in some cases a family member.[38] In sub-Saharan Africa, for example, the estimates of births occurring without trained attendants is higher at 58%; in Asia it is 47% (Figure 1-9).

Are all women in resource-poor settings "stuck" at home, where they lack emergency care and commonly have inadequate means of timely transport for a mother and/or newborn to a referral facility should birth not be normal? Some are indeed. However, many stay home because this is what they know and want. WHO acknowledges that families, especially in rural and resource-poor settings, still choose homebirth with a traditional midwife or a relative, precisely because of their immediate availability, the lower cost, and their adherence to culturally valued practices (WHO, 1996).[39]

There is a fundamental challenge in matching policy to practice. Lessons can be learned from the natural childbirth movement:

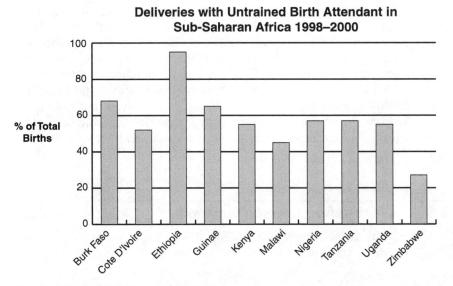

Source: DHS ORCMACRO, Inc DHS 1998–2000

FIGURE 1-9 In Africa, many women still deliver at home with an untrained attendant.

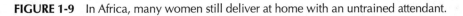

namely, that there is value to keeping birth normal and natural. Institutionalization of childbirth has the disadvantages of introducing procedures and restrictions, some not scientifically evidenced based, as to who may accompany the laboring woman, what she may eat or drink during labor, and in what position she must labor and deliver. Routine episiotomy and other medical procedures and practices have become the norm. These practices may actually keep rural and traditional families away from hospitals even when they need to be there for medical reasons.

Appropriate Technology in Birth and Breastfeeding

In 1985, only four years before the publication of the 1989 joint statement on *Protecting, Promoting, and Supporting Breastfeeding,* a technical meeting was convened in Fortaleza, Brazil, by the Pan American Health Organization (PAHO) and WHO European Office, wherein experts provided consultation and review of the evidence and developed "recommendations for appropriate technology in birth."[40] These recommendations highlighted the need

for respectful care and noninvasive interventions during childbirth (Box 1-4). After review of the evidence, specific recommendations included encouraging the mother's mobility in labor and
choice of position for delivery, abolishing routine episiotomies,
discouraging routine artificial rupture of membranes, questioning
high rates of oxytocin induction of labor, and suggesting that
facility cesarean section rates above 10–15% were not justifiable.
Recommendations, which supported breastfeeding, included initiation of breastfeeding and no separation of mother and baby.

BOX 1-4   Fortaleza Recommendations

WHO Joint Interregional Conference on Appropriate Technology for Birth

Fortaleza, Brazil, 22–26 April, 1985

General Recommendations:

1. Health ministries should establish specific policies about
   the incorporation of technology into commercial mar-
   kets and health services.
2. Countries should develop the potential to carry out
   cooperative surveys to evaluate birth care technology
3. The whole community should be informed about the
   various procedures in birth care, to enable each woman
   to choose the type of care she prefers.
4. Women's mutual aid groups have an intrinsic value as
   mechanisms for social support and the transfer of
   knowledge, especially with relation to birth.
5. Informal perinatal care systems (including traditional
   birth attendants), where they exist, must coexist with the
   official birth care system and collaboration between
   them must be maintained for the benefit of the mother.
   Such relations, when established in parallel with no concept of superiority of one system over the other, can be
   highly effective.
6. The training of people in birth care should aim to
   improve their knowledge of its social, cultural, anthro-
   pological and ethical aspects.
7. The training of professional midwives or birth attendants should be promoted. Care during normal preg-

nancy and birth, and following birth, should be the duty of this profession.

8. Technology assessment should be multidisciplinary and involve all types of providers who use the technology, epidemiologists, social scientists, and health authorities. The women on whom the technology is used should be involved in planning the assessment as well as evaluating and disseminating the results. The results of the assessment should be fed back to all those involved in the research as well as to the communities where the research was conducted.

9. Information about birth practices in hospitals (rates of Cesarean section, etc.) should be given to the public served by the hospitals.

10. The psychological well being of the new mother must be ensured not only through free access to a relation of her choice during birth but also through easy visiting during the postnatal period.

11. The healthy newborn must remain with the mother, whenever both their conditions permit it. No process of observation of the healthy newborn justifies a separation from the mother.

12. The immediate beginning of breastfeeding must be promoted, even before the mother leaves the delivery room.

13. Countries with some of the lowest mortality rates in the world have Cesarean section rates under 10%. Clearly there is no justification in any geographic region to have more than 10–15% Cesarean section births.

14. There is no evidence that Cesarean section is required after a previous transverse low segment Cesarean section birth. Vaginal deliveries after a Cesarean should be encouraged wherever emergency surgical capacity is available.

15. There is no evidence that routine intrapartum electronic fetal monitoring has a positive effect on the outcome of pregnancy. Electronic fetal monitoring should be carried out only in carefully selected medical cases (related to high perinatal mortality rates) and in induced labor. Countries where electronic fetal monitors and qualified staff are available should carry out investigations to select specific groups of pregnant women who might benefit from electronic fetal monitoring. Until such time

continued

Box 1-4 continued

       as results are known, national health services should abstain from purchasing new monitoring equipment.

16. There is no indication for pubic hair shaving or a predelivery enema.

17. Pregnant women should not be in a lithotomy position during labour or delivery. They should be encouraged to walk about in labour and each woman must freely decide which position to adopt during delivery.

18. The systematic use of episiotomy is not justified. The protection of the perineum through alternative methods should be evaluated and adopted.

19. Birth should not be induced for convenience, and the induction of labour should be reserved for specific medical indications. No geographic region should have rates of induced labour over 10%.

20. During delivery, the routine administration of analgesic or anesthetic drugs that are not specifically required to correct or prevent a complication in delivery should be avoided.

21. Normally rupture of the membranes, as a routine process, is not scientifically justified.

There was a logical overlap among the 1985 evidence-based Fortaleza recommendations on appropriate technology in birth, the 1987 SMI call for a clean, safe delivery, and the 1989 joint statement on protecting, promoting, and supporting breastfeeding and the special role of maternity services. Yet, at the global policy and implementation level, these links have largely not occurred.

Medical Education and Separation of Obstetrics and Pediatrics

Academic and professional specialties can disrupt the mother-baby dyad. In most medical and nursing education hospitals, in both developing and developed countries, education on childbirth is increasingly the domain of obstetrical specialists and care of the newborn is under the jurisdiction of pediatricians. With the expansion of these separate medical specialties, responsibility for infant feeding and breastfeeding has fallen largely to the pediatricians. This separation of the mother and the newborn within the medical and nursing training institutions may point to some of the difficulties discussed in this book in identifying the connections between birthing practices and breastfeeding. Midwifery training in general is an exception to this separation and a professional midwife is taught to provide care to the healthy woman and baby during pregnancy, birth, lactation, and intra-conceptionally. It is indeed fortunate that WHO has identified the midwife as the "most appropriate and cost effective type of health provider to be assigned to the care of normal pregnancy and normal birth, including risk assessment and recognition of complications."[41] As the research is reviewed, it becomes clear that, in models where midwives are truly the gatekeepers of keeping birth normal, breastfeeding remains the most intact as well.[42-47] The role that midwives have and must continue to play in the protection of the continuum will be emphasized as specific childbirth interventions are reviewed in this book.

Innocenti Declaration 1990: A Call to Action

In 1990, WHO, UNICEF, and other key health funding agencies convened a high-level consensus meeting in Innocenti, Italy. The goal of this meeting was to gather together global policy makers, including Ministers of Health, to form a consensus to set operational targets for "protection, promotion, and support of breastfeeding." The outcome was the Innocenti Declaration, which sets a global goal for optimal maternal and child health and nutrition. The role women play is highlighted:

> Efforts should be made to increase women's confidence in their ability to breastfeed. Such empowerment involves the removal of constraints and influences that manipulate perceptions and behavior towards breastfeeding, often by subtle and indirect means. This requires sensitivity, continued vigilance, and a responsive and comprehensive communications strategy involving all media and addressed to all levels of society. Furthermore obstacles to breastfeeding within the health system, the workplace and the community must be eliminated.[48]

The call is there within the Innocenti Declaration to address "obstacles within the health system" by improving birthing practices and optimizing breastfeeding outcomes. It is not too late to begin. Now is the time to re-link care of the mother during her labor and delivery to early newborn care and breastfeeding outcomes. This will restore to mothers something that they have lost with the move towards medicalized hospital births: a sense of high self-esteem, of being in control, and of empowerment throughout their pregnancy, birth, and breastfeeding experience (Figure 1-10).

Return to Normal

Solid scientific evidence shows that returning to birthing practices that preserve normalcy can accomplish many things: faster, easier births; healthier, more active and alert mothers and newborns; and mother-baby pairs physiologically optimally ready to breast-feed. In addition to the quantifiable evidence is the cumulative wisdom of women who still know that normal, natural childbirth and breastfeeding go together. This wisdom comes from village women in Indonesia, Ethiopia, and Guatemala who fear referral to the hospital in childbirth because of the inhumane and invasive treatment they may receive. This wisdom comes from the natural childbirth pioneers in the 1970s in the United States who fought for and won back the right to nonmedicalized birth. This wisdom comes from the brave young first-time mother in 2003 who dares to defy her peers, labors without epidural anesthetic, and discov-

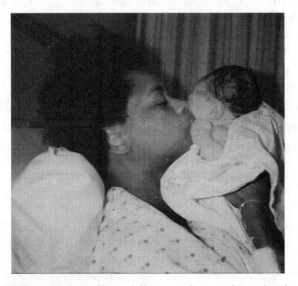

FIGURE 1-10   Ella joyfully greets her newborn daughter immediately after birth. She is the first to hold and kiss her.   *Photo by Janis Fox-Davis, 1982.*

ers the power in pushing out her own baby, lifting this precious gift right up into her own arms, and putting the baby to breast.

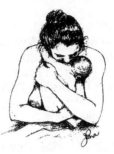

References

1. Mitford J. 1992. *The American Way of Birth*. New York: Dutton.
2. Smith M., and Holmes L.J. 1996. *Listen To Me Good*. Columbus, Ohio: Ohio State University Press.
3. Ashford JI. 1986. *Mothers and Midwives: A History of Traditional Childbirth*. Booklet and slide set. Self-published and out of print
4. Dick-Read G. 1944. *Childbirth Without Fear: The Principles and Practice of Natural Childbirth*. New York: Harper.
5. Karmel M. 1959, 1981, 1983. *Thank You, Dr. Lamaze*. New York: Harper Colophon Books.
6. White M. 2002. Personal communication.
7. Tompson M. 2002. Personal communication
8. Cahill M.A. 2001. *Seven Voices, One Dream*. Schaumburg, IL: La Leche League International.
9. La Leche League International. 1958. *The Womanly Art of Breastfeeding*, 1st ed. Franklin Park, Illinois: La Leche League International.
10. La Leche League International. 1963. *The Womanly Art of Breastfeeding*, 2nd ed. Franklin Park, Illinois: LLL International.
11. La Leche League International. 1972. *On Nursing the Newborn...How Soon?* Information Sheet No. 20. Revised April 1972.
12. White M., and Thornton C. 1978. *Together, and Nursing. From Birth*, La Leche League International. Information Sheet No. 20. Revised January 1978.
13. La Leche League International. 2002. *LLL/I Annual Report, 2001–2002*. Schaumburg, Illinois.
14. La Leche League International. 1985. *Purpose and Philosophy*. Publication No. 5. La Leche League International, Schaumburg, Illinois.
15. La Leche League International. 1991. *The Womanly Art of Breastfeeding*. Thirty-fifth Anniversary ed. New York: Penguin Books.

16. Gaskin I. 1977. *Spiritual Midwifery,* 1st ed. Summertown, TN: The Book Publishing Company.

17. Klaus M. and Kennell J. 1982. *Parent-Infant Bonding.* Saint Louis: C.V. Mosby Co.

18. Freeman M. 1979. Giving Family Life a Good Start in the Hospital. *Am J Mat Child Nursing* 4(1):51–54.

19. Li R, CDC Epidemiologist, 2002. Personal Communication. Maternal Child Nutrition Branch, Nutrition and Physical Activity Division, Center for Disease Prevention and Control (Data read from National Survey of Family Health–1956–87 and Ross Laboratories–1988–90.)

20. Davis-Floyd R. 1992. *Birth As an American Rite of Passage.* Berkeley and Los Angeles: University of California Press.

21. Cohen N.W. 1991. *Open Season: Survival Guide for Natural Childbirth and VBAC in the 90's.* New York: Bergin and Garvey.

22. Mitford J. 1992. *The American Way of Birth.* New York: Dutton.

23. Pfeufer-Kahn R. 1995. *Bearing Meaning: The Language of Birth.* Urbana and Chicago: University of Illinois Press.

24. Data for graph from various sources: 1970–88 data from Center for Disease Control. 1995. *Rates of Cesarean Delivery–United States 1993 MMWR* 44(15):303–307.R; 1989–94 data from NCHS Hospital Discharge Surveys; 1989–94 data from National Vital Statistics Reports (1995–2001).

25. United States Department of Agriculture. Women, Infants and Children Website. *www.fns.usda.gov/wic/Breastfeeding/bfleghistory.HTM.*

26. American Academy of Pediatrics. 1997. Policy Statement: Breastfeeding and the Use of Human Milk (RE9729). *Pediatrics* 100(6):1035–1039.

27. Gross L. 2002. Statistical report for the 2002 examination. Falls Church, VA: International Board of Lactation Consultant Examiners.

28. Ryan A. 1997. The Resurgence of Breastfeeding in the United States. *Pediatrics* 99(4): e12. (Data based on Ross Laboratories Mothers' Survey.)

29. Declercq E.R., Sakala C., Corry M.P., Applebaum S., and Risher P. 2002. *Listening to Mothers: Report of the First National U.S. Survey of Women's Childbearing Experiences.* New York: Maternity Center Association. October 2002, *www.maternity.org/listeningto mothers/results.html.*

30. Sharp K. 2002. Personal communication (with permission to use Internet text from the Lactnet, Tuesday, November 05, 2002 5:54 PM).

31. Magalhaes, Rebecca. 2002. Personal communication.

32. Smith, Linda J. 2002. Personal communication.

33. Center for Disease Control. 1999. Achievements in Public Health, 1900–1999: Healthier Mothers and Babies. *MMWR* 48(38):849–858.

34. WHO/UNICEF (Joint Statement). 1989. *Protecting, Promoting, and Supporting Breast-Feeding: The Special Role of Maternity Services.* Geneva: WHO.

35. UNICEF, 2003. "Report on Progress on the WHO/UNICEF BABY FRIENDLY HOSPITAL INITIATIVE (BFHI)." Presented by Miriam Labbok at the "WHO Consultancy on the Global Strategy on Infant and Young Child Feeding" February 10, 2003.

36. WHO. 1994. *Mother-Baby Package: Implementing Safe Motherhood in Countries.* Geneva: WHO. WHO/FHE/MSM/94:11.

37. WHO. 1996. *Care in Normal Birth: A Practical Guide.* Geneva: WHO. WHO/FHE/MSM/96:24.

38. WHO. 1998. *World Health Day Safe Motherhood 7 April 1998.* Information Kit, Division of Reproductive Health, WHO, Geneva.

39. WHO. 1996. *Care in Normal Birth: A Practical Guide.* Geneva: WHO. WHO/FHE/MSM/96:24.

40. WHO. 1985. *Joint Interregional Conference on Appropriate Technology for Birth, Fortaleza Brazil, 22–26 April, 1985.* (Report number ICP/MCH 102/m O 2(S) 0175V 10 June 1985).

41. WHO. 1996. *Care in Normal Birth: A Practical Guide.* Geneva: WHO. WHO/FHE/MSM/96:24.

42. Janssen P.A., Lee S.K., Ryan E.M., et al. 2002. Outcomes of Planned Home Births versus Planned Hospital Births after Regulation of Midwifery in British Columbia. *CMAJ* 166(3):315–323.

43. Korte D. 1992. Infant Mortality: Lessons from Japan. *Mothering Magazine.* Winter: 83–89.

44. Tyson H. 1991. Outcomes of 1001 Midwife-Attended Home Births in Toronto, 1983–1988. *Birth* 18(1):14–19.

45. Fisher C. 1990. A midwife's view of the history of modern breast-feeding practices. *Int J Gynecol Obstet.* 31(Suppl.1):47–50.

46. Rooks J., et al. 1989. Outcomes of Care in Birth Centers: The National Birth Center Study *New Engl J Med.* 321:1804–1811.

47. Haire D. 1981. Improving the Outcomes of Pregnancy through Increased Utilization of Midwives. *J Nurse Midwifery.* 26 (1):5–8.

48. UNICEF. 1990. *Innocenti Declaration on the Promotion, Protection, and Support of Breastfeeding.* 1 August 1990, Florence, Italy. UNICEF Nutrition Cluster. New York.

CHAPTER 2

EVIDENCE-BASED PRACTICE IN PERINATAL CARE

"Not everything that counts can be counted and not everything that can be counted, counts."

Albert Einstein, physicist

Evidence-Based Care: What Evidence Really Counts?

There is currently great emphasis on grounding medical practice on sound research evidence. According to research scientists, the most credible research on health care outcomes is from randomized, controlled, double-blind clinical trials. What does this mean? *Randomized* studies include study subjects who have been chosen in a statistically random manner from a defined population, without any bias in selection. *Controlled* studies use samples of subjects who are studied with a new approach or intervention; these subjects are "matched" with a sample of similar subjects from the same population who will continue with the routine standard of care as a "control" group. Often criteria are set for subjects—they must all be healthy, must be first-time mothers, or must be of a similar socioeconomic class.

Whenever the research design allows, studies are even stronger if subjects are *blinded*, meaning that the subjects themselves do not know who is receiving the intervention and who is not. *Double-blinded* means that neither the subject nor the researcher knows who is getting the intervention and who is the control; thus the study results are evaluated with the greatest degree of freedom from bias. For example, if one is testing the effectiveness of a new drug, the study group receives the experimental drug and the control group receives a *placebo*, or inert substance, packaged as if it were the drug being tested. Each subject is blind as to who is receiving what, and the study can further be double-blinded if the person assessing the drug effectiveness is not aware of which group received the study drug. Blinding serves to lessen or eliminate bias on the part of either subject or researcher towards the outcome of the intervention and the conclusions drawn from the study.

Challenges of Research on Childbirth and Lactation

What if the researcher is looking at a childbirth intervention such as introducing the presence of a support person at the bedside of the laboring mother, and then assessing the impact on one outcome, for example length of labor? Here it is possible to randomize and control study subjects, but not to introduce blinding because it will be obvious which mother has a support person at the bedside. In studying labor and childbirth, there are always potentially *confounding factors*, or factors that can confuse the results or reduce the "strength" of the conclusions. In this example, the study population could, for example, be defined as only first-time mothers with normal pregnancies, and who had normal deliveries of single term infants. However, there are still many possible confounding factors in this "defined" study sample: the mother's preparation for childbirth or lack thereof, the size and position of the baby, the use or non-use of pain medicine in labor, the amount of time the mother walks or stays sedentary during labor, and so on. In spite of these limitations, such studies have produced convincing evidence that continuous support in labor has a positive effect on length of labor.

Researchers have looked further and have asked if labor support can influence breastfeeding. In this research there are certainly additional confounding factors such as length of pushing, whether or not an episiotomy was performed, or whether or not routine newborn procedures were done immediately after birth. These additional actions can confound matters and make conclusions less convincing. Chapter 3 of this book more closely examines this research on the impact of continuous support in labor on childbirth outcomes, including length of labor, method of delivery, and need for other obstetrical interventions. A randomized controlled trial approach becomes difficult when studying populations of pregnant mothers, trying to match subjects so that they are identical or nearly identical, and minimizing confounding factors. In research on childbirth, subjects generally come from "convenience samples" of pregnant mothers who at the time of the study agree to be subjects and are willing to be randomized into the control or study group and who continue to fit the criteria for admission as a subject (that is, they did not develop confounding complications during labor and delivery). However, pregnant mothers are human beings, with all their preconceptions, past and present life events, and the physiologic and cultural forces that come to bear during childbirth. This makes rigorous study of childbirth much more difficult than, for example, testing the effectiveness of a new drug.

Cochrane Pregnancy and Childbirth Database

The most significant contribution to the evidence-based approach to perinatal care comes from a project started decades ago by Iain Chalmers and other colleagues, who began to organize a register of controlled clinical trails. Rigorous criteria were utilized for acceptance of this research. In addition to published clinical research, in the early years of establishing this database, some 40,000 obstetricians in 18 countries were polled for unpublished data that might be considered as protocols for care. The first major publication that came from this effort was a two-volume, 1500 page book called *Effective Care in Pregnancy and Childbirth* in which standards for perinatal care were supported by rigorous research.[1]

Two other user-friendly sources for this information also became available. One is *A Guide to Effective Care in Pregnancy and Childbirth*, which summarizes the analysis of the clinical trials into a format that readily provides guidance for perinatal care.[2] The other is the electronic database established for general reference in 1995 and regularly updated as The Cochrane Library.[3] These systematic, up-to-date summaries constitute reliable evidence of the benefits and risks of health care and are intended to help policy makers and clinicians make sound practical decisions. The Cochrane database is available to anyone who pays the subscription fee and has access to electronic mail. The reviews are full-text articles reviewing the effects of health care research. They are highly structured and systematic, with evidence included or excluded on the basis of explicit quality criteria to minimize bias. Data are often combined statistically (with meta-analysis) to increase the power of the findings of numerous studies that are too small to produce reliable results individually.

WHO *Reproductive Health Library*

The World Health Organization (WHO) has utilized the Cochrane database to provide health care planners and clinicians in developing countries with the most current information on reproductive health care. The *Reproductive Health Library* (RHL) is updated annually, and the most current issue[4] contains 70 Cochrane reviews and corresponding commentaries. These reviews are grouped by topic, and they present policies and practices that have been proven through appropriate scientific methods. In addition, commentary is provided on evidence of provider and user satisfaction and on the feasibility and cost-effectiveness of the practice in different settings.

Jose Villar, the RHL coordinating editor, writes: "The WHO Reproductive Health Library seeks not only to prevent the introduction of unsubstantiated health care practices into programs, but also to replace the practices that have been demonstrated to be ineffective or harmful with those based on best available evidence."[5] Subscriptions to the RHL are free to developing countries, and, since 1997, a computer format (on CD-ROM) has been available with key articles, studies, reviews, corresponding commentaries, and practical recommendations for clinical care. Even teaching videos can be uploaded from this disc onto a computer.

The RHL No. 5 has a section that categorizes six levels of evidence, called the "Effectiveness Summaries for Decision-making." These levels, based on the rigor of the studies, are categorized as follows:

1. Beneficial forms of care
2. Forms of care likely to be beneficial
3. Forms of care with a trade-off
4. Forms of care of unknown effectiveness
5. Forms of care likely to be ineffective
6. Forms of care likely to be harmful

Based on Cochrane reviews, practices are categorized within these six levels. Examples from RHL No. 5 of practices rated by strength of the evidence are listed in Box 2-1.

Box 2-1   Examples of practices categorized by level of evidence, from WHO RHL No. 5, 2002

1. Beneficial forms of care:
   - External cephalic version at term reduces breech delivery and cesarean section rates.
   - Social support during labor in busy, technology-oriented settings reduces the need for pain relief and is associated with a positive labor experience.
2. Forms of care likely to be beneficial:
   - Social support during labor in busy, technology oriented settings could lower caesarean section rates, number of infants with low Apgar scores (< 7 at 5 min) and duration of labor.
   - Kangaroo-mother care method of skin-to-skin contact in low-birth-weight infants is associated with reduced likelihood of illness at six months and exclusive breastfeeding at discharge from hospital.
3. Forms of care with a trade-off:
   - When compared to intermittent auscultation of the heart rate, routine electronic fetal heart rate monitoring during labor is associated with fewer neonatal seizures, similar long-term infant outcome, but increased caesarean section rates.
   - Intramuscular prostaglandins are effective in reducing blood loss in the third stage of labor but their safety is uncertain and their costs are prohibitive in under-resourced settings.
4. Forms of care of unknown effectiveness:
   - Using postural [position] maneuvers to convert breech to vertex presentation on incidence of breech delivery is unknown.
   - The effectiveness of kangaroo-mother care method in reducing neonatal and infant mortality and exclusive breastfeeding at one or six months is unknown.
5. Forms of care likely to be ineffective:
   - Early amniotomy (breaking of the bag of waters) during labor in reducing caesarean section rates
   - Routine electronic fetal monitoring during labor for low-risk pregnancies.
   - Routine intubation at birth in vigorous term meconium-stained babies to prevent meconium aspiration syndrome.

continued

Box 2-1 continued

6. Forms of care likely to be harmful:
   - A policy of routine episiotomy to prevent perineal/vaginal tears compared to restricted use of episiotomy.
   - Forceps extraction instead of vacuum extraction for assisted vaginal delivery when both are applicable is associated with increased incidence of trauma to the maternal genital tract.

Other Resources for Evidence-Based Maternity Care

A Guide to Effective Care in Pregnancy and Childbirth, now in its third edition has established an approach to evidence-based practice and forms the basis for medical obstetrical protocols for the United Kingdom and Canada. It draws from the steadily accumulating research in the Cochrane pregnancy and childbirth database. The third edition, with 50 chapters and over 500 pages, provides a wealth of recommendations on state-of-the-art perinatal care. Of the seven authors, six are physicians and one is a nurse. Two authors are Australian, two are British, two are Canadian, and one is South African. Notably absent are authors from the United States, and no funding for any of these editions has ever come from a U.S. source.

Chapter 46 of the third edition is on breastfeeding. The introduction to this chapter mentions that social and psychological support in labor "may increase the likelihood that mothers will breastfeed their babies successfully." The next sentence reports that "sedative and analgesic drugs given during labor can alter the behavior of the newborn infant, and compromise its crucial role in the initiation of lactation." These are essentially the only links made to childbirth practices and breastfeeding outcomes. The next section in the chapter covers "Antenatal preparation," and the third section is on "Early versus later suckling." Omitting any discussion on intrapartum management in this chapter essentially mirrors the same omission in the Ten Steps to Successful Breastfeeding presented in Chapter 1. Given the overall scope of this book, it is unfortunate that research analysis has not been provided for studies that have associated childbirth practices with breastfeeding.

Another publication, *Managing Complications in Pregnancy and Childbirth: A Guide for Midwives and Doctors,* presents state-of-the-art practice standards for facility-based clinicians in resource-poor settings and countries.[6] This manual has a companion manual for primary health care level providers. The preface states: "The interventions described in these manuals are based on the latest available scientific evidence. Given that evidence-based medicine is the standard on which to base clinical practice, it is planned to update the manual as new information is acquired." It is reassuring to see that many obstetrical practices such as having a support person in labor, discouraging routine episiotomy, and early initiation of breastfeeding are included as recommended standards of care.

Evidence-Based Breastfeeding Practices

The Ten Steps to Successful Breastfeeding (see Chapter 1) evolved from research evidence available in 1989, and forms the basis of the UNICEF/WHO Baby Friendly Hospital Initiative. Nearly a decade later, another document, *Evidence for the Ten Steps to Successful Breastfeeding*, provides additional and more current evidence for the implementation of BFHI in maternity facilities.[7] This publication takes each of the Ten Steps and reviews the credible research that supports each step. The authors state that their review methodology included only published studies and "as far as possible only randomized controlled ('experimental') studies and controlled studies where allocation was systematic or when a 'before and after intervention' design was used ('quasi-experimental')." The document summarizes all studies reviewed in a table format, complete with a description of research methodology, interventions, results, and major and minor limitations of each study. The chapter on Step Four, "Help mothers initiate breastfeeding within a half-hour of birth," includes reviews of eleven studies that support the evidence for this step. Of note is the concluding section of this chapter, "Other Outcomes," in which five more studies are cited that suggest a negative effect on breastfeeding if the mother receives labor analgesia. In all five studies reviewed, the labor drug was meperidine (Demerol and Pethidine). One additional study is mentioned, which showed "that the perception of severe pain was significantly lower in a group of women who had supportive companionship when compared to a group that had routine care. Evidence for the effect of other methods [of pain relief] is not available."[8] It is unfortunate that the authors do not mention here that the same supportive companionship study looked at breastfeeding and mothering outcomes at six weeks postpartum. These outcomes included exclusive breastfeeding rates, reported feeding difficulties, and reported ease of mothering, with significant results showing a positive correlation between support in labor and exclusive breastfeeding and mothering behavior at six weeks after the birth. The authors' conclusions in this chapter include "routine use of pethidine should be minimized," but this recommendation has not made it into the BFHI assessment process to date.

A symposium on The Nature and Management of Labor Pain was held in 2001 in New York. One of the papers prepared for this meeting reviewed a large number of clinical trials on parenteral opioids (narcotics given intravenously or by injection) for labor pain relief. Many childbirth interventions and outcome variables were analyzed in this paper but the authors were unable to analyze breastfeeding because none of the studies has included it as an outcome. The authors' discussion section begins:

> Although 48 trials contributed some data to this review, the findings are not easy to interpret. For some of the outcomes, no information was available from any of the clinical trials, *most notably for breastfeeding and mother-infant bonding* [author's emphasis]. In some trials there was no usable data on the pre-specified primary outcomes, neonatal resuscitation (reported in 15% of trials), and maternal satisfaction with pain relief.[9]

The Politics of Research

The academic and clinical division between obstetrics and pediatrics, in which the former claims domain over pregnancy, childbirth, and general breast health and the latter claims domain over the newborn and breastfeeding, may partially account for the research gap that exists. Literature searches linking the keywords of "birth intervention" and "breastfeeding" reveals a dearth of literature in which the primary research question asks how a certain birth intervention is linked to breastfeeding outcomes. Is this just an oversight or is it intentional? Dr. Michel Odent comments on two types of epidemiological research: circular research and cul-de-sac research.[10] In circular research, studies are repeated and continued beyond the point of reasonable doubt, or in other words, there is a tendency to test the same question again and again. Cul-de-sac research includes research about issues that "despite the publication of this research in authoritative medical or scientific journals, ... are shunned by the medical community and the media. Cul-de-sac epidemiological studies are not replicated, even by the original investigators and they are rarely quoted after publication." Odent's article concludes:

> A pessimistic analysis focusing on the difficulties of epidemiology may inspire the simplistic conclusion that politically correct research leads to "circular epidemiology" and that politically incorrect research leads to "cul-de-sac epidemiology." An optimistic analysis would stress that it is possible to break through the dead end of a cul-de-sac and open an avenue. In other words the limits of political correctness are not immutable. Let us welcome break-through epidemiology.

Taken out of the context, Odent's observations on epidemiological research may seem very abstract. However, he was for years a practicing obstetrician in France where he and midwife colleagues pioneered in promoting a model of maternity care that recognized the importance of protecting the mother from interference during and immediately after childbirth. After retiring from practice, Odent continued writing and speaking about the need to "humanize" birth, most notably in his books *The Nature of Birth and Breastfeeding* (1992) and *The Scientification of Love* (1999). Although his work is widely read by midwives, natural childbirth activists, and families who are seeking nonmedicalized childbirth, it has not been mainstreamed into modern obstetrical or pediatric textbooks. Perhaps linking birth and breastfeeding is "politically incorrect?" Perhaps it would be crossing lines delineated by medical specialties and reinforced by lack of evidence-based research. Dr. Odent is very clear on this issue: "On the day when human societies return to their role as protectors of the mother and baby instead of meddling in their relationship, then humanization will naturally follow."[11]

Early Research: Oxytocin or "The Love Hormone"

Some of the most instructive research on childbirth and lactation was done nearly half a century ago, preceding the natural childbirth awakening and the resurgence of breastfeeding. Psychologist Niles Newton and her spouse, Michael Newton, an obstetrician, identified and wrote about the psycho-physiologic aspects of lactation, stressing the interrelationship between a mother's sense of well-being and her subsequent breastfeeding success.[12]

In pioneering research spanning from 1948 through 1979, the Newtons published widely on the subject, drawing their conclusions first from animal studies documenting that cows will not "let down" their milk easily when a cat is put on their backs or when they are given injections of adrenaline.[13,14] They reproduced this finding for human lactation with a sample size of one human subject (Niles herself, breastfeeding her seven-month-old infant) by showing that milk let-down is fairly easily influenced by outside events. They showed that noxious stimuli such as immersion of feet in ice water, painful toe pulling, or math calculations with electric shock after wrong answers, would inhibit breast milk ejection. They also linked milk ejection to plasma oxytocin levels.[15,16]

Niles Newton (see Figure 2-1) continued over the next two decades to examine the reproductive hormone oxytocin and its role in coitus, labor, delivery, and lactation, and in 1971 she published one of a series of articles on the interrelationship between sexual intercourse, childbirth, and lactation. She proposed that these reproductive events share at least three characteristics: 1) they are based on closely related neurohormonal reflexes; 2) they are sensitive to environmental stimuli, being easily inhibited in their early stages; and 3) they all, in certain circumstances, trigger care taking.[17]

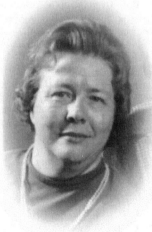

FIGURE 2-1   Niles Newton in the mid 1970s.   Photo used with permission of Edward R. Newton and Karen L. Newton.

As Newton developed her thesis, she suggested that this inhibition of milk let-down or the milk ejection reflex was built into mammalian psychophysiology as a safeguard from milk stealing. She points out the key role played by oxytocin in human sexual excitement and orgasm, in the normal progress of labor and delivery, and in the milk ejection reflex during breastfeeding. Oxytocin secretion can be inhibited by adrenaline or the fight or flight reaction if danger approaches, in which case mammals, including humans, would be vulnerable to attack or danger. Newton theorized that oxytocin secretion could be protected by a negative feedback system that would 1) block the trancelike state that occurs during deep sexual arousal, 2) stop the progress of labor until safer surroundings are found, or 3) inhibit milk let-down until mother and baby can safely feed.

This classic work on oxytocin supports a premise of this book, namely that initiation of lactation will be most successful if the entire reproductive process is preserved in a setting of emotional and social support free from anxiety, fear, and danger. In spite of what is known about oxytocin's role in parturition and lactation, the increasingly technological and invasive approach of modern obstetrics often works against the flow of normal labor, delivery, and immediate optimal bonding.

Technology: Too Much and Too Little Can Be Dangerous

In developing countries and resource-poor settings, there may not be modern technology and often not even essential obstetric and newborn medicines, equipment, and staff skilled in their use. There is often an unsafe environment that includes inadequate, uncomfortable, or unclean facilities; lack of privacy; and/or a shortage of staff who can or will provide a caring, respectful, family-centered childbirth environment. While lack of medicines and equipment is a serious situation that may take longer to correct, privacy, the provision of respectful care, and a climate of family support does not cost much and could go far to provide the safe environment needed for normal birth (Figure 2.2).

What would Niles Newton have said about the drive to have randomized controlled clinical studies point the way for all perinatal care? As a sample size of only one, she might never have bothered to immerse her feet in ice water while she was breastfeeding her infant in order to measure the impact this had on milk let-down. We know, however, that as a social scientist Niles Newton also

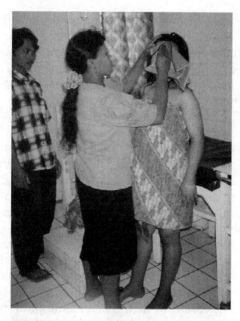

FIGURE 2-2 A small district hospital in Central Java implemented mother-friendly evidence-based care including allowing family members to be present in the labor ward and encouraging the mother to walk and drink fluids freely during labor. *Photo by Mary Kroeger, 1997.*

valued the incredible body of undocumented knowledge and practice, by speaking with indigenous peoples, midwives, mothers, and newborns, who spoke to her with their behavior.

The Cochrane database regularly reviews and rates research studies and meta-analyses of these studies, from which best practices in obstetrical and neonatal care can and should be standardized. Yet in many settings, notably in the United States, the research seems not to have taken hold, practices for which there is clear-cut evidence are still being ignored, and others that are actually harmful are still all too common.[18] Linda Smith, a lactation consultant of over 25 years, observes, "There is no smoking gun, but clearly there is something happening during medicalized birth that is affecting the way babies suck."[19] Clinical experience, case reports, and sometimes what "just works" must guide our care and advice until there is additional research (Figure 2-3).

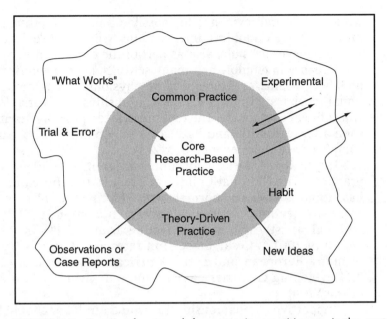

FIGURE 2-3   Practice framework for maternity practitioners. In the center or core there is evidence-based practice (where it exists), and it should be used. In the next ring there is theory-based practice, things commonly done or with a basis in general understanding of biology, but no corroborating research as yet. The third ring contains what is being done without any careful analysis, but continues as practice because "it works" or someone else says it works. In the outer ring are new ideas or experiments in process. As more research is developed, any given practice in the outer or middle ring can move towards the center. If it moves to the core, we should incorporate it, and if it is proved ineffective or harmful we should discontinue it.   (Source: Smith, 2002)[20]

Breaking Through the Cul-de-Sac

This book attempts to close the research gap between childbirth and lactation management by analyzing research that has been categorized as highly significant by rigorous reviews as well as research that may have some weaknesses in design but still provides valuable information. The complexity of labor may confound the ability to prove causality, so the challenge is to probe deeper into these suspected causes and relationships rather than to ignore them. The work of principle investigators who are nurses and midwives is frequently highlighted as their research design often gets closer to the unanswered questions. Chapter by chapter, individual childbirth interventions will be examined along with the research evidence for possible links to or influences on breastfeeding. Childbirth interventions will be looked at alone and, whenever possible, also as part of the cascade of events that is the reality in childbirth in many settings. Even the most normal of labors begins as a complex of physiologic, anatomic, emotional, social, and cultural interrelationships and variables that will influence its course. The first breastfeed optimally occurs very soon after childbirth, and its success may reflect the normalcy or complexity of those events (Box 2-2).

The United States is not alone in ignoring evidence-based practices. The National Childbirth Trust in the United Kingdom has noted a drop in "normal birth" (defined as birth without cesarean section, assisted delivery, induction of labor, or regional anesthesia) with a decline from 57.2% in 1992 to 44.4% in 2001.[21] Cesarean section rates are at an all-time high in many European and Latin American counties (see Chapter 8). Developing countries have all too quickly adopted the ways of the West.

Supportive companionship for women in labor should be the norm in every maternity ward in the world. This is not an expensive intervention; in fact it has been shown to be cost-effective in reducing expensive medical interventions. There is no excuse for routine episiotomy, still the most common surgical incision in global obstetrics, because the evidence shows clearly that this is actually a harmful routine practice. As the Innocenti Declaration mandates, maternity hospitals everywhere can and should be Baby Friendly Hospitals.

Box 2-2 Cascade of Interventions. Normal labor can become a cascade of interventions, which can affect breastfeeding outcomes.

Evidence shows that lack of continuous support in labor, especially among young primagravidas (first-time mothers), can create poor coping behavior, exacerbate anxiety and pain, and slow labor progress. Slowed labor may necessitate "augmentation" with intravenous oxytocin to bring stronger, more regular labor contractions, and may require the woman to be confined to bed with a decrease in her ability to walk or even to change position in labor. In some settings, oxytocin drip protocols require frequent electronic fetal monitoring, thus further limiting the woman's movements. With the strengthened contractions from the oxytocin drip, the mother may become more anxious and the pain may increase, leading to need for pain medication. Narcotic analgesia can lead to slowed and/or dysfunctional labor and thus, ironically, the oxytocin dose must be increased to further strengthen labor. Labor medication can also affect the newborn's ability to initiate breastfeeding. There is literature that associates regional/spinal epidural anesthesia for pain relief in labor to higher rates of instrumental and surgical deliveries, and some studies associate these interventions with breastfeeding difficulties. Often, either as routine care or when the labor becomes "abnormal or prolonged," a mother may have all oral fluids withheld "in case" she might need a cesarean section. Yet unless the mother remains well hydrated and nourished, the keto-acidosis (breakdown of the mother's fat stores) produced by prolonged withholding of food may also hinder labor progress and lead to the fetus becoming additionally stressed.

If these interventions do not move the labor along at the prescribed rate (in some settings this is based on the partograph, an international labor guide that mandates a centimeter dilatation per hour), then the decision is made for a cesarean section. Or, if the mother is at the second stage of labor (complete dilation, when pushing may begin), there may be an assisted, instrumental delivery with forceps or vacuum extraction.

The cascade continues. Poorer breastfeeding outcomes (both initiation and duration) are linked to long labors and to surgical or assisted deliveries. Because many of these interventions precede operative or surgical delivery, it is difficult to know which factors are linked to breastfeeding difficulty. If an assisted or surgical delivery was performed for fetal distress, the baby may not be in a condition for early initiation of breastfeeding. If it was an assisted or surgical delivery for obstructed labor (also know as "failure to progress"), the mother may be exhausted, under the influence of labor and/or surgical anesthesia, in pain, or all three. Frequently, both the mother and the newborn may be in poor condition for bonding and early breastfeeding and will be separated after birth. Even when both mother and baby are fine, newborn procedures are often performed immediately after the delivery thus interfering with uninterrupted skin-to-skin contact with the mother.

Summary Points for Protecting the Mother-Baby Continuum:

- There is a major research gap in current research that examines the impact of childbirth practices on breastfeeding outcomes.
- Randomized controlled clinical trials are not ethically possible for many childbirth interventions and this level of research cannot be seen as the only valid measure of evaluating childbirth and breastfeeding outcomes.
- Evidence-based care, while being seen as the highest standard for practices, is not reflected in many current obstetric interventions and practices.

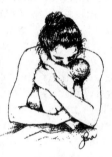

References

1. Chalmers I, Enkin MW, and Keirse M. 1989. *Effective Care in Pregnancy and Childbirth,* Oxford: Oxford University Press.
2. Enkin M, Keirse M, Renfrew M, Neilson J. 2000, *A Guide to Effective Care in Pregnancy and Childbirth,* Third edition, Oxford: Oxford University Press.
3. Cochrane Library. 2000. Update Software Ltd, Oxford, England, *http://www.update-software.com.*
4. World Health Organization (WHO). 2002. *Reproductive Health Library* No. 5, 2002 Geneva: WHO/RHR/02 1.
5. Villar J, Gülmezoglu AM, Khanna J, Carroli G, Hofmeyr GJ, Schulz K, Lumbiganon P. 2002. Evidence-Based Reproductive Health In Developing Countries, *WHO Reproductive Health Library* (No. 5), Geneva: WHO/RHR/02.
6. WHO, UNFPA, UNICEF, World Bank. 2000. *Managing Complications in Pregnancy and Childbirth: A Guide for Midwives*

and Doctors. World Health Organization, Department of Reproductive Health and Research, WHO/RHR/00.7.

7. WHO. 1998. *Evidence for the Ten Steps to Successful Breastfeeding.* Geneva: WHO/CHD/98.9.

8. Hofmeyr GJ, Nikodem VC, Wolman W, et al. 1991. Companionship to modify the clinical birth environment: Effects on progress and perception of labour, and breastfeeding. *Brit J of Obstet Gynecol* 98:756–764.

9. Bricker L and Lavender T. 2002. Parenteral opioids for labor-pain relief: A systematic review. *Am J Obstet Gynecol* 186:S94–109.

10. Odent M. 2000. Between circular and cul-de-sac epidemiology. *Lancet* 355 (9212):1371.

11. Odent M. 1992. *The Nature of Birth and Breast-feeding.* Westport, Connecticut: Bergan and Garvey.

12. Newton N. 1987. In Introduction to: *Newton on Breastfeeding: Reproductions of Early Classic Works by Niles Newton with Michael Newton and Others.* Rev. ed. 1990. Seattle, Washington: Birth and Life bookstore.

13. Ely F, Petersen WE. 1941. Factors involved in the ejection of milk *J Dairy Science* 24:211.

14. Petersen WE, Ludwick TM. 1942. The hormonal nature of factors causing let-down of milk. *Federation Proceedings* 1:66.

15. Newton M and Newton N. 1948. The let-down reflex in human lactation. *J Pediatr* 33:693–704.

16. Newton M and Newton N. 1950. Relation of the let-down reflex to the ability to breastfeed. *Pediatrics* 5:726–733.

17. Newton N. 1971. Trebly Sensuous Woman. *Psychology Today,* 71 (July):68–71.

18. Declercq ER, Sakala C, Corry MP, Applebaum S, Risher P. 2002. *Listening to Mothers: Report of the First National U.S. Survey of Women's Childbearing Experience.* New York: Maternity Center Association, *www.maternity.org/listeningtomothers/results.html.*

19. Smith, Linda J. 2003. Personal communication.

20. Smith LJ. 2002. "Core Concepts" diagram first introduced during a *Lactation Consultant Exam Preparation Course* taught in May 1998.

21. Hotelling B. 2002. Personal Report on the Normal Labour and Birth First Research Congress, Lancashire, UK, October 2002.

CHAPTER 3

LABORING WITH A SUPPORT PERSON AND BREASTFEEDING

"Research has shown bright lights on what women have always known."
Robin Lim, midwife and author, 2000

Chapter 1 discussed the shift of childbirth in industrialized countries from the home to the hospital. This change brought with it the exclusion of family members from this life event. In homebirth, family members traditionally provided the main support for women during labor, birth, and postpartum, but when birth moved to hospitals, the laboring woman was separated from her family and whisked off to the "sterile" maternity ward. Her partner and family were expected to wait for news of the baby's birth in a waiting room, and their first view of the baby was most often through the window glass of the newborn nursery.

Background

With the advent of the natural childbirth movement in Europe in the 1950s, both Dr. Fernand Lamaze in France[1] and Dr. Grantly Dick-Read in England[2] wrote of the importance of help and attention to the laboring woman. By the 1960s and early 1970s, the natural childbirth consumer movement in the United States brought forth the demand for family participation in labor and birth. This change came easily in some settings and was hard won in others. Gradually maternity ward doors opened, first to the spouse or partner of the laboring woman, and eventually to extended family and friends.[3,4] Especially difficult was shifting the policy to allow the family in the delivery room (see Box 3-1).

Box 3-1   Handcuffed to the Wife in Labor

Retired California nurse-midwife Carole Hagin recalls her days as a childbirth educator and labor coach in the mid 1960s before she began attending births at home in her San Francisco East Bay community. One large HMO hospital where many of her clients delivered had strict policies prohibiting anyone other than an approved trained labor "coach" to accompany the woman during labor and delivery. One couple tried all means to convince the hospital administration to permit the husband to be with his wife in the delivery room, but with no success. He was with his wife in the labor room, but when she was ready to go to the delivery room he quickly handcuffed himself to his wife's wrist and had to go into the delivery with her. Hagin recalls that he was successful both in making his point and being at the delivery of his baby!

Hagin reports another incident at the nearby county hospital when a husband wanted to be present at the birth of his baby and the staff refused him. After persisting in his request he was finally "allowed" to be present in the delivery room, but only with the arrangement that he was strapped into a wheelchair that was wheeled by the nurse next to the delivery table. The rigid policy of no family member present at a woman's birth finally changed officially at this hospital, Hagin recalls, only when the wife of a staff doctor wanted him present with her in the delivery room.

Source: Carole Hagin, RN, CNM, 2003[5]

It is now the norm for a laboring woman to have family with her in maternity hospitals in most industrialized countries. However, in much of the nonindustrialized world, the woman who has her baby in a hospital, whether by plan or due to referral, still labors alone with only the support that is provided by maternity staff. In resource-poor countries, hospitals are often understaffed and maternity care providers are overworked, and underpaid, and thus may be unable or unmotivated to provide continuous emotional support to their laboring patients. Typically, the family must wait outside the maternity ward, even when the mother was brought in for emergency reasons and the family may have paid (for them) huge sums of money to get the woman to the hospital for care. This exclusion of her family may bring fear to the mother in labor and may separate her from a family member who may be able to translate from a local dialect or give information about the early course of her labor.

Until very recently, in most of Eastern Europe and the former Soviet Union, separation of a mother from her family during childbirth was extreme. The family—even the husband—could not even enter the maternity hospital during the labor, birth, or even postpartum, and they did not see mother or baby until she was discharged, usually seven days after delivery (Figure 3-1). The policy for this isolation of the mother was set in Soviet doctrine, and this practice was prevalent across all of Eastern Europe and

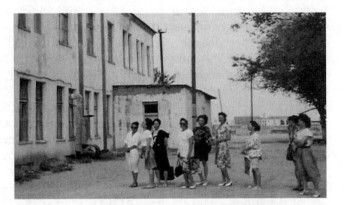

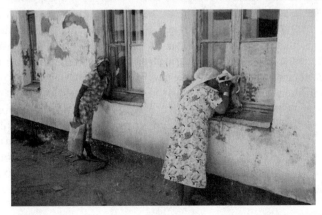

FIGURE 3-1 Former Soviet Union: routine exclusion of family support, Atyrau Oblast, Western Kazakhstan. Top: Eager family members wait outside a maternity hospital to catch a glimpse of the new baby if the mother can hold the baby up to the window. Bottom: New grandmothers try to give advice to their daughters about baby care through closed windows of a post-partum ward. *Photos by Mary Kroeger, 1994.*

the Soviet Union. These rigid policies remained in place even as the natural childbirth movement evolved in Europe and the United States. Since the mid 1990s there have been dramatic changes in some maternity policies in the former Soviet Union, and the practice of isolating the maternity patient from her family is gradually disappearing. Through intensive training programs incorporating evidence-based care, maternity policies are encouraging a support companion for women in labor.[6]

Labor Support: Better Birth Outcomes, Breastfeeding, and Mothering

Common sense suggests that a woman would labor more calmly and effectively with someone supporting her during childbirth. Yet the need for evidence to prove this has led to several important studies in the last two decades. These studies have looked at the impact on various birth outcomes of the presence at the bedside of a laboring woman of a supportive relative, health provider, or lay labor companion or doula.* These studies have varied as to the cohort characteristics, the type of labor companion, whether this support was continuous or intermittent, and also as to the specific outcomes examined. All have looked at labor length and mode of delivery. Several have examined the use of specific labor management interventions such as oxytocin augmentation and the use of pain medication. Others have looked at support and subsequent condition of the infant (fetal distress, APGAR scores, and transfer to neonatal intensive care), at the psychosocial impact on the new mother, and a few have examined the impact on breastfeeding.

In 1980, the first randomized controlled clinical study was conducted on the effect of labor support on perinatal problems in Guatemala City by a team that included Roberto Sosa, John Kennell, and Marshall Klaus.[8] This study looked at 32 low-risk primagravida women in labor who were supported by a lay doula and 95 controls. Women were removed from the study if they had prolonged labor, fetal distress, need for oxytocin augmentation, or cesarean section. As an incidental result, the authors were surprised to find that far fewer of their doula-supported group had to be excluded from the study because of any of the aforementioned

---

Doula is from the Greek meaning "woman caregiver of another woman" and in these studies refers to an experienced labor companion who provides non-medical support, both emotional and physical, to a woman throughout labor and delivery (Klaus and Klaus, 1993).[7] In these studies not all labor companions were trained doulas, but rather relatives or motivated community-based women.

complications. Overall, their findings were that the supported group of mothers had significantly shorter labors: 8.8 hours on average versus 19.3 hours in the control group. The supported mothers were awake more after delivery, and also stroked, smiled at, and talked to their babies significantly more.

Following this work, the same authors looked directly at maternal and infant morbidity in a much larger randomized control study at the same Guatemalan hospital. They found that compared to the control group (N = 249), the supported group (N = 168 after exclusions) benefited in the following ways: fewer C-sections, less need for oxytocin augmentation, shorter labors, and fewer perinatal complications overall.[9]

Kennell and Klaus brought essentially the same research question to a large American hospital.[10] In a randomized controlled study, two experimental groups and one control group of approximately 200 each were sought among healthy primagravidas. One experimental group was assigned a trained doula and the other experimental group was assigned an observer who was present in the room but who neither touched nor spoke to the laboring woman. Their results are dramatic, confirming their earlier findings and showing that even the presence of a neutral observer has an impact on birth outcomes (Table 3-1).

Meta-Analyses on Impact of Labor Support

Three meta-analyses on the data on labor support have been performed to date.[11–13] The first, in 1994, was included in the Cochrane review. A comprehensive review and discussion of these meta-analyses has subsequently been done by Scott, Klaus, and Klaus.[14] These authors analyzed twelve randomized controlled clinical trials, using the selection criteria of subjects being healthy primagravidas who entered the study in early labor (less than 4 cm dilation). The selected trials represent hospital care in four European countries, two states in the United States, and two each from Canada, Guatemala, and South Africa. Their review divides the discussion of findings across the 12 studies into obstetrical findings and postpartum findings.

Key obstetrical findings were that women with labor support had their duration of labor significantly reduced by up to an average of 98 minutes when compared to the control group. The supported women had significantly less need for pain medication, oxytocin augmentation, forceps, vacuum extraction, and cesarean section. A distinction is made in the type of labor support across the studies reviewed, and the overall conclusion is that continuous support is

TABLE 3-1 Effects of Emotional Support During Labor

Outcome	Supported (n = 212)	Observed (n = 200)	Control (n = 204)	P Value
Narcotic analgesia	21.7%	28%	25.5%	no difference
Epidural anesthesia	7.8%	22.6%	55.3%	<.0001
Oxytocin augmentation	17%	23%	43.6%	<.0001
Duration of labor (mean)	7.4 hours	8.4 hours	9.4 hours	= .0001
Cesarean delivery	8%	13%	18%	= .009
Forceps delivery	8.2%	21.3%	26.3%	<.0001
Prolonged hospitalization of newborn	10.4%	17%	24%	<.001
Sepsis evaluation	4.2%	9.5%	14.7%	<.001
Maternal fever	1.4%	7%	10.3%	= .0007

Adapted from Kennell J, Klaus M, et al (1991). Continuous emotional support during labor in a U.S. hospital. A randomized controlled trial. *Journal of the American Medical Association* 265(17):2197–2201. Used with permission.

more effective than intermittent support. Continuous support is defined as "the labor attendant remaining with the mother without interruption, except for toileting, from shortly after admission in labor, throughout labor and until birth of the infant."[15]

Logically, a mother who has had a shorter, less exhausting, less invasive labor and birth will be more ready and eager to bond with and breastfeed her newborn. Thus, the positive obstetrical outcomes seen in these studies on support in labor are of keen interest as they stand by themselves. The additional postpartum findings discussed in this review confirm the validity of this inference. Eight of the 12 trials explored postpartum effects associated with support in labor. In the earliest studies in Guatemala[8] mothering behavior was also studied by observing the new mothers through a one-way mirror in the first 25 minutes after leaving the delivery room. The mothers in the experimental group were more likely to be smiling, talking to, and stroking their babies than were the nonsupported mothers.

In 1991, a South African randomized controlled study on support in labor investigated similar obstetrical outcomes with less remarkable findings in differences in length of labor or need for pain medication.[16] The cesarean section rates in both study and control groups were very similar and were appropriate for an urban inner-city referral hospital: 12% in the study group and 14% in the control groups, respectively. In their discussion, the authors suggest that the less dramatic findings in their study, compared to the similar Guatemalan and U.S. studies done by Kennell and Klaus, et al., were likely due to several factors; first, the companionship was less effective; second, the medical interventions were less frequent; and third, the "adverse" environmental effects were less intense in the South Africa setting, thus creating less room for noting improvement. For example, epidural anesthesia was not available at all to the South African subjects.

The Hofmeyr research additionally focused on the psychosocial effects of labor support, and baseline psychosocial variables were measured in both groups before labor and then again at one day postpartum and six weeks postpartum. At 24 hours after delivery, assessment of the new mother's current anxiety, perceived pain, ability to cope in labor, and the number of activities already undertaken with the baby was significantly more favorable in the supported group. At six weeks postpartum, the supported group's anxiety scores remained significantly lower, and self-esteem scores were higher. Parenting behaviors were markedly more positive in the supported group: 45% of the supported group found "becoming a mother easy" compared to only 11% of the control group. As for breastfeeding, 51% of the study group were exclusively breastfeeding compared to 29% of the controls; 81% of the supported group

TABLE 3-2   Mothers' Responses at Six Weeks Postpartum on Infant Feeding

Mother Reports	Support Group (n = 74)		Control Group (n = 75)		P value
Is exclusively breastfeeding	38	(51.4%)	22	(29.3%)	0.01
Has a flexible feeding interval	60	(81.1%)	35	(46.7%)	0.0001
Has feeding problems	12	(16.2%)	47	(62.7%)	0.0001
Finds mothering easy	33	(44.6%)	8	(10.7%)	0.001
Baby has poor appetite	0	(—)	19	(25.3%)	0.001

Adapted from Hofmeyr GJ, et al. (1991).[16]

reported having "flexible" feeding schedules compared to the 47% in the control group; and none of the supported group felt her baby had a "poor appetite" compared to 25% of the mothers in the control group (Table 3-2). These findings are striking and certainly suggest that perception of how a mother coped with labor may be linked to how successfully she breastfeeds and how she perceives coping with new motherhood.

A study not included in the three meta-analyses has also documented the positive impact of labor support on breastfeeding. In a similarly designed randomized controlled study in Mexico City with an urban middle-class population, there was a positive effect on breastfeeding with the doula group as well as a reduction in the length of labor.[17] Exclusive breastfeeding rates at one month postpartum in both groups, however, were not high—12.3% in the supported group compared to 7.5% in the control—and there is a strong cultural norm in Mexico City to feed with a mix of breast milk and formula. It is also worth noting that the epidural anesthesia rates for both groups, supported and controlled, were very high at 88% and 87%. It is possible that this extensive and routine use of epidural anesthesia may have had a confounding effect on the overall success with exclusive breastfeeding (See Chapter 6).

Another study looked at several factors affected by the use of doulas in a large health maintenance organization (HMO) in California.[18] Findings included that the presence of a doula significantly reduced the rate of epidural anesthesia and that mothers were more likely to report their birth experience as "good" and to feel they had coped well in labor. No differences were seen in breastfeeding, both groups had a 95% early initiation of breastfeeding rate, and 90% in the doula group and 87% in the control group were still breastfeeding at four weeks postpartum. The authors note that for all mothers in the HMO study institutions there is a comprehensive breastfeeding education program and postpartum breastfeeding support for all patients, and that most who choose to breastfeed do so successfully.

Childbirth Support in Resource-Poor Settings

Few studies to date have examined the impact of labor support in a more traditional population or a resource-poor setting. One randomized controlled clinical trial in such a setting was conducted in Botswana, Southern Africa.[19] In this study, patients in the study area came from a background in which they normally delivered at home with a traditional birth attendant and with support from female family members. Conducted at the largest referral hospital, 109 women meeting the criteria of being healthy, nulliparous (no previous deliveries), and in early, uncomplicated labor were chosen at random. All of the women were ethnic black *Batswana* with a mean age of 19. The women in the study cohort each had a chosen female relative untrained in any special doula techniques to remain with her throughout labor and delivery. The control cohort had routine care by the staff. Outcomes were dramatic. The supported group had a significantly higher number of normal spontaneous deliveries (91% compared to 71%), half as many cesarean sections, one fourth as many vacuum extractions, and significantly less need for anesthesia, amniotomy (breaking the amniotic membranes to hasten labor), or oxytocin augmentation (Table 3-3).

Breastfeeding outcomes were not examined in the Botswana study, but the vast majority of women in Botswana (at the time of this publication) initiated breastfeeding.[20] The authors posit that the experimental mothers "suffered less stress, pain, anxiety, and tension" as a result of having a relative at the bedside and all evidence suggests that these mothers, 91% of whom had normal vaginal delivery, would have been optimally ready to immediately initiate breastfeeding. An unexpected outcome was that staff midwives responded spontaneously to the study by inviting companions to be with women not in the study. The referral hospital in

TABLE 3-3   Botswana Study on Impact of Support by Female Relative on Delivery Method and Other Labor Interventions

Outcome	Supported Group (n = 53)	Control Group (n = 56)	P Value
Spontaneous vaginal delivery	91%	71%	0.03
Vacuum extraction	4%	16%	0.03
C-section	6%	13%	0.03
Analgesia	53%	73%	0.03
Amniotomy	30%	54%	0.01
Oxytocin in first stage of labor	13%	30%	0.03

Adapted from Madi B, et al. (1999).[19]

the capitol city of Botswana is not markedly unrepresentative of referral hospitals throughout sub-Saharan Africa. Findings are particularly important because the obstetrical outcomes are consistently better in a group of first-time mothers who simply had the support of a female relative.

Health Care Providers As Barriers to Change

Staff midwives and doctors are not always as open to innovative change as was the staff in the Botswana study. In Zambia, a recent study was conducted to examine the views of both mothers and staff in both urban and rural maternities concerning the introduction of social support during labor.[21] The majority of the 84 mothers interviewed were in favor of being attended by a supportive companion. On the other hand, many of the 40 health staff interviewed cited hospital policy as reasons why this would not be possible, and some worried that the support persons would "interfere" with their work. Most staff, however, acknowledged that emotional support could be helpful and that first-time

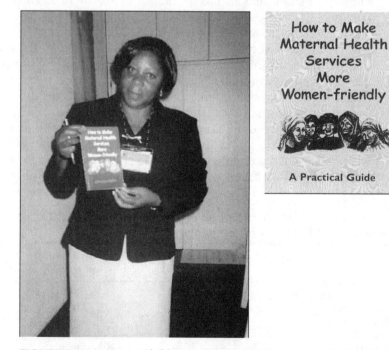

FIGURE 3-2   Maureen Chilila, principal midwifery tutor at University Teaching Hospital Lusaka, Zambia, holds a practical guide for health workers on how to improve maternity care.   *Photo by Mary Kroeger, 2002.*

mothers would especially benefit. Plans were then made to change the policy in order to introduce companionship in labor in Zambian maternity wards (See Figure 3-2). With the help of international funders, Zambian midwives were trained and they are now asking mothers to identify a "support person" from their family and friends during the antenatal period. This person accompanies the mother to the antenatal clinic, receives health education along with her, and comes with her in labor to the maternity unit.[22] The constraints that still exist include lack of privacy in general labor wards—curtains are needed between beds. However, the presence of a support person is becoming more common in the main university teaching hospital and in 23 health centers throughout Zambia (Figure 3-3).

Program Implications

The essential ingredients of the labor support companions in the research described are that they are usually female and are continuously present with the laboring women. They do not provide any medical care, but rather provide praise, encouragement, reassurance, comfort measures, physical contact (massage, rubbing, hand holding), and explanation on progress and what is transpiring in labor. Also of note is that in the Guatemala, South Africa, and Botswana studies, the support persons were laypersons without any special training. For resource-compromised areas, this fact lends assurance that the introduction of female support into labor wards need not involve expensive training programs, but rather involves maternity staff willing to embrace these support people as an unofficial but very valuable part of the childbirth team. This cost-effective intervention could provide a great service to the commonly understaffed maternity hospitals in resource-poor countries and settings, and an increase in normal deliveries saves money otherwise spent in costly medicines and surgical procedures.

There are many programs in Europe, the United States, and Australia that train labor support people or doulas, and these care providers have already become integrated into the routine maternity care in many hospitals. Also, husbands and partners still rightfully want to be present at the birth of their children, and the restrictions on extended family being present—even children—has loosened considerably in the last decade (Figure 3-4).

In any setting, if the labor support intervention can be continued into early postpartum care and can be combined with early and effective initiation of breastfeeding, it is likely that breastfeeding outcomes would be positively affected as well.

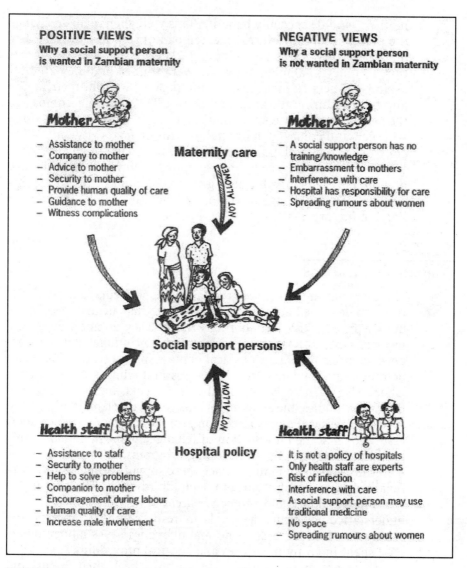

FIGURE 3-3 Views of mother and health staff on involvement of social support persons in Zambian maternities.   Figure 1 from Journal of Midwifery & Women's Health, v 46(4): 232, Maimbolwa MC et al.: "Views on involving a social support person during labor in Zambian maternities." © 2001 American College of Nurse-Midwives.

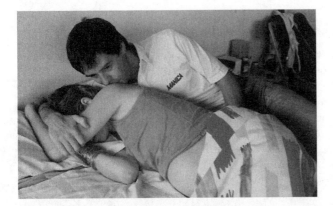

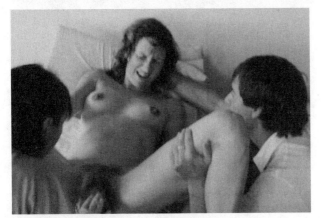

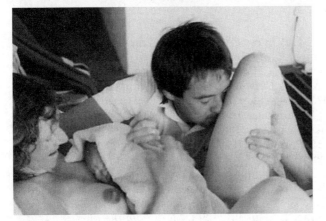

FIGURE 3-4   Birth of Luke.   Steve touches and supports Maggie:
Top: smooching in early labor; Middle: encouragement while pushing;
Bottom: joyful tears and touch after delivery.   *Photos by Robert Armstrong,
Swaziland, 1989.*

Summary of Points for Protecting the Mother-Baby Continuum
- Compelling evidence documents that continuous female labor support reduces the need for many labor interventions and improves birth outcomes. This effect is especially significant for primiparas (first-time mothers).
- Growing evidence suggests that breastfeeding and mothering are positively affected by labor support.
- In spite of the clinical evidence for and cost effectiveness of introducing companionship in labor as the standard of care, maternity hospitals in the developing world most have not yet adopted this intervention.

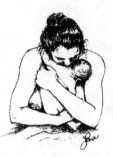

References

1. Lamaze F. 1954. *Painless Childbirth: The Lamaze Method.* Chicago: Contemporary Books, Inc.
2. Dick-Read G. 1944. *Childbirth Without Fear: The Principles and Practice of Natural Childbirth.* New York: Harper.
3. Arms S. 1975. *Immaculate Deception, A New Look at Childbirth in America.* Boston: San Francisco Book Company/Houghton Mifflin Books.
4. Karmel M. 1959, rev. 1981. *Thank You, Dr. Lamaze.* Harper and Row, Publishers, Inc.
5. Hagin C. Personal communication, January 2003.
6. Chalmers B, and Porter R. 2001. Assessing Effective Care in Normal Labor: The Bologna Score. *BIRTH* 28 (2): 79–82.
7. Klaus M, Kennel J, Klaus PH. 1993. *Mothering the Mother.*: Addison Wesley Publishing.
8. Sosa R, Kennell J, Klaus M, et al. 1980. The effect of a supportive companion on perinatal problems, length of labor, and mother-infant interaction. *N Engl J Med* 303:597–600.

9. Klaus M, Kennell J, Robertson SS, Sosa R. 1986. Effects of social support during parturition on maternal and infant morbidity. *Br Med J* 293(6547):585–587.

10. Kennell J, Klaus M, et al. 1991. Continuous emotional support during labor in a U.S. hospital. *JAMA* 265(17):2197–2201.

11. Hodnett ED. 2001 Caregiver support for women during childbirth. In *The Cochrane Library,* Issue 3. Oxford: Update Software (original analysis Neilson JP, Crowther CA, Hodnett ED, et al, 1994 in Issue 2. Oxford: The Cochran Collaboration).

12. Scott KD, Berkowitz G, Klaus M, et al. 1999. A comparison of intermittent and continuous support during labor: A meta-analysis. *Amer J Obstet Gynecol* 180(5):1054–1059.

13. Zhang J, James W, Bernasko MB, et al. 1996. Continuous labor support from labor attendant for primiparous women: A meta-analysis. *Obstet Gynecol* 88:739–744.

14. Scott K, Klaus PH, Klaus M. 1999. Review: The obstetrical and postpartum benefits of continuous support during childbirth. *J Women's Health Gender-Based Med* 8(10):1257–1264.

15. Kennell J, Klaus M, McGrath S, et al. 1991. Continuous emotional support during labor in a US hospital. *JAMA* 265(17):2197–2201.

16. Hofmeyr GJ, Nikodem VC, Wolman W, et al. 1991. Companionship to modify the clinical birth environment: Effects on progress and perception of labour, and breastfeeding. *Brit J of Obstet Gynecol* 98:756–764.

17. Langer A, Campero L, Garcia C, et al. 1998. Effects of psychosocial support during labour and childbirth on breastfeeding, medical interventions, and mothers' well being in a Mexican public hospital: A randomized clinical trail. *Brit J of Obstet Gynecol* 105:1056–1063.

18. Gordan N, Walton D, McAdam E, et al. 1999. Effects of providing hospital-based doulas in health maintenance organization hospitals. *Obstet Gynecol* 93:422–426.

19. Madi BC, Sandall J, Bennett R, et al. 1999. Effects of female relative support in labor: A randomized controlled trial. *Birth* 26(1):4–8.

20. Madi BC. 2002. Personal communication.

21. Maimbolwa M, et al. 2001. Views involving a social support person during labor in Zambian maternities. *J Midwifery and Women's Health* 46(4):226–234.

22. Maimbolwa M, and Chilila M. University Teaching Hospital, Lusaka, Zambia. Personal communications, 2003.

CHAPTER 4

MATERNAL POSITION IN LABOR, BIRTH, AND BREASTFEEDING

"Our women keep their dresses on and deliver in the kneeling position. The baby comes easy and the mother can see it right away. This is how we have always done it."

Alfonsa Ico, Mayan midwife, Belize, 2002

Is the mother's mobility and position during labor and birth related to breastfeeding outcomes? To explore this connection in this chapter, as with the chapters that follow on hydration, medication, and mode of delivery, it will be necessary to piece together what research exists, and at the same time reflect back on the cascade of events that occur when labor becomes prolonged, requires medication, or complications develop. If mobility and the upright position in labor facilitates faster, less painful, and more physiologic delivery, surely these conditions influence a mother's or newborn's readiness to breastfeed.

Background

Like the need for supportive companionship, the need to walk and move around during labor and to stay upright during delivery is empirical wisdom to laboring women worldwide (Figure 4-1). In the photo essay, *Mothers and Midwives: A History of Traditional Childbirth,* numerous ancient and modern works of art and sculpture from around the world *depict* women at the moment of birth.[1] The early images and art pieces are of women in the upright position: standing, squatting, or semi-sitting and usually attended by

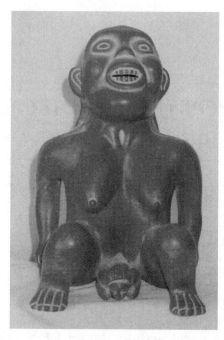

FIGURE 4-1 Birth Goddess:
Tiacoilteuti. Aplite Valley
Mexico, 1325–1521 (Reproduc-
tion). *Photo courtesy of Jenna
Houston.*

others. As the pictorial essay moves into the nineteenth and twentieth centuries, the images taken from medical texts show the
change in birthing position from upright to supine.

Medical practitioners in Europe began to use forceps in the late
1500s, and began performing delivery in the supine position. Dr.
Joseph DeLee formally introduced the lithotomy position (on the
back with legs in stirrups) to modern American obstetrics in the
early 1900s in his textbook, *Principles and Practice of Obstetrics.*
This book, first published in 1913, strongly advocated for sedation
in labor, routine episiotomy, and use of forceps.[2] DeLee's influence
radiated rapidly to the rest of the western world, where women were
put to bed to labor, kept there, and delivered on their backs, often
even with restraints on arms and legs. In the United States and
Europe, it wasn't until the advent of the natural childbirth movement in the 1960s and 1970s that the desire to be out of bed in labor
and upright in at least a semi-sitting position to deliver was again
insisted on by women in childbirth (Figure 4-2).

Physicists would argue that a 5–10 pound object (a baby)
needing to be expelled through a muscular yet elastic passage
(the birth canal) would benefit from the force of gravity added to
the intrinsic forces of pushing (uterine contractions and pushing

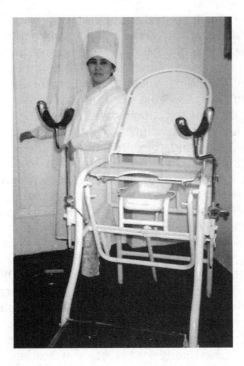

FIGURE 4-2 In many countries delivery chairs are very high, uncomfortable, and even frightening. Sometimes mothers fear their baby will drop on the floor at time of delivery. *Photo by M. Kroeger, Kazakhstan 1994.*

by the mother). Dr. Caldeyro-Barcia in Uruguay began investigating the effects of position in labor on uterine contraction patterns and fetal outcomes as early as 1960.[3] In 1979, he carried out a now classic study of the influence of maternal position on the duration of labor.[4] He found that "vertical" mothers had 36% shorter first stages of labor on average than "horizontal" women did, the vertical mothers reported less pain, and their infants were less likely to have marked molding of the head after delivery. One of the most important findings in this study was that physiologic pushing in the upright position, with a woman pushing 5 to 6 seconds and breathing before she pushed again, led to less fetal hypoxia and acidosis (fetal distress) as measured by cord blood gases after birth.

Position in the First Stage of Labor

There are no randomized controlled trials on position in the first stage of labor and birth outcomes, much less on breastfeeding outcomes. It was shown by Caldeyro-Barcia and colleagues that delivery of the mother in the dorsal (supine) position can lead to compression of the uterus on the great vessels of the mother and thus can compromise fetal oxygenation.[5] Most current midwifery textbooks, childbirth education classes, and doula training curricula describe in detail the advantages of a woman being free to move around in labor and choose a position that feels right for her. Perhaps the biggest consideration for this discussion is how a mother feels about her own freedom to choose when and how much to move around, sit, stand, rock on hands and knees, shower or bathe, or assume any other positions. Often a mother will instinctively assume a position that favors faster, more effective labor. Midwives know that if the fetal head is presenting in an occiput posterior (OP) position (the back of the baby's head is facing towards the mother's back), then assuming a hands and knees position can often help the fetal head to spin to a more favorable occiput anterior position and make for an easier delivery (see Figures 4-3 through 4-5). Labor with a persistent OP presentation can be more painful to mothers due to the increased pressure on the sacrum, thus leading to a higher chance that pain medication may be required. Labor may be prolonged, leading to the need for oxytocin augmentation, perhaps additional medication, and often an assisted delivery or cesarean section. All of these latter interventions, as later chapters will discuss, may be linked to interference in early, effective breastfeeding.

Box 4-1   "Culture Lag" is still lagging...

The recent *Listening to Mothers* survey in the United States of childbearing experiences among 1583 women who responded to telephone interview or electronic mail survey reported that 71% of women who were admitted to maternity facilities did not walk around *even once* after regular contractions began. The primary reason given for not walking was that they were "connected to things" (67%). Other reasons reported for staying in bed were pain "medications that made them unable to support themselves" (32%), being told by the care provider not to walk around (28%), and grogginess from pain medication (20%). The percentage who chose to stay in one place was 20%.

Source: Declercq ER, Sakala C, Corry MP, Applebaum S, Risher P. 2002.

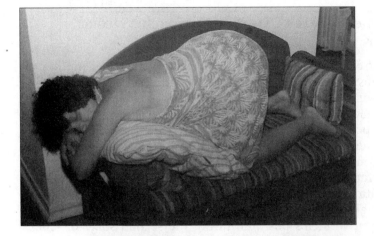

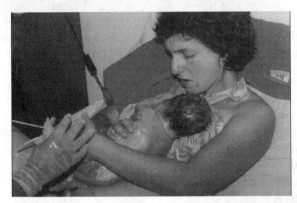

FIGURES 4-3, 4-4, AND 4-5 Deborah had a persistent occiput posterior presentation as she began labor, and she spontaneously adopted this posture (top) during contractions. The baby rotated and delivery was accomplished easily, with breastfeeding initiated within minutes of Xavier's birth (right). *Photos by Martin Butcher, 1992.*

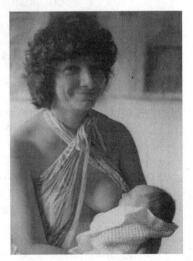

Meta-Analyses on Women's Position During the Second Stage of Labor

Since the early studies that looked at getting women in labor off their backs, obstetric care in the United States and Europe has adapted to the growing evidence and now encourages ambulation in labor and birth in more upright positions. Many hospitals now have beds that include position controls and can convert into modified birthing stools, and many have squat bars. Birth centers usually encourage delivery in the position of the women's choice, and most midwives are comfortable with delivery in many different positions.

Gupta and Nikodem reviewed 18 randomized (or quasi-random allocation) clinical trials for an article in the Cochrane Library on women's position during the second stage of labor.[7] They compared the use of all upright and lateral positions to the supine or lithotomy positions. Outcomes measured included numerous maternal, fetal, and neonatal outcomes. Breastfeeding success was not included as an outcome in any of the studies. Maternal findings included an association between the use of upright or lateral position and reduced length of and pain during the second stage, small reductions in instrumental deliveries, reduction in episiotomy, but an increase in second-degree lacerations (tears to the perineum). There were no significant neonatal outcomes. Their conclusions from this review are that there are some advantages to upright position for the mother and that until there is more rigorous clinical evidence for the advantages of one position over another, mothers should be free to make "informed choices" about position for delivery.

Researcher Bias in Results and Conclusions

Not included in the meta-analysis is a cohort study conducted by two midwives and one physician, which compares outcomes from squatting in the second stage of labor to semi-recumbent positions.[8] Data were obtained by chart review of patient delivery records from two hospitals in the northeastern part of the United States. Although charts were examined retrospectively, the authors term the study prospective because the outcomes were not known at the onset of chart review. A random sampling of 1000 charts allowed selection of study and control groups, both including primiparas and multiparas with similar normal obstetric history and socioeconomic status. Findings were that squatting women (n = 200) had faster second stages, required less labor stimulation with oxytocin, and showed a trend toward fewer assisted deliveries than did the semi-

TABLE 4-1   Length of Second Stage (Pushing) and Delivery Method by Position

Variable	Second Stage (in mins)	Spontaneous Delivery	Assisted Delivery
Squatting primip (n = 105)	71	92%	8%
Semi-recumbant primip (n = 53)	95	83%	17%
Squatting multip (n = 92)	19	98%	2 %
Semi-recumbant multip (n = 47)	32	98%	2%

*Adapted from Golay et al. (1993). Table 1 from Golay J., The Squatting Position for the Second Stage of Labor: Effects on Labor and on Maternal and Fetal Well-Being. Birth 20:2 June 1993 © 1993 Blackwell Scientific Publications, Inc. Used with permission.

recumbent mothers (n = 100) in the control (see Table 4-1). The squatting group also had fewer episiotomies and severe lacerations (Table 4-2). There was no statistical difference in complications of the third stage of labor (delivery of placenta) or in infant complications as measured by Apgar scores.

It is interesting to compare this study to another somewhat similar study done about the same time by researchers in Bombay, India.[9] These clinicians questioned whether the squatting position, compared to their usual practice of supine delivery, increases the efficiency of labor and birth and also is not detrimental to maternal and infant. This study was a randomized controlled prospective study and patients were randomly assigned to study and control groups of 100 women each, including both primiparas and multiparas. There is no indication in the study design that the

TABLE 4-2   Perineal Integrity by Birth Position and Parity (Third and Fourth Degree not Included)

Variable	Intact	1st degree laceration	2nd degree laceration
Squatting primip (n = 98)	43.9%	27.5%	28.6%
Semi-recumbant primip (n = 17)	24%	29%	47%
Squatting multip (n = 86)	56%	30%	14%
Semi-recumbant multip (n = 32)	44%	28%	28%

*Adapted from Golay et al. (1993). Table 2 from Golay J., The Squatting Position for the Second Stage of Labor: Effects on Labor and on Maternal and Fetal Well-Being. Birth 20:2 June 1993 © 1993 Blackwell Scientific Publications, Inc. Used with permission.

wishes of the mother herself were a consideration in clinical management. Those in the squatting group were "kept ambulatory" during labor and "were made to squat on the delivery cots" for the second stage. Those in the supine group were "kept in supine position throughout labor." Results included measuring the length of the first and second stage and maternal trauma as defined as any laceration, extension of episiotomy, or cervical tears.

These authors found that both first and second stages were dramatically diminished in the ambulatory/squatting group, with the primiparas experiencing a 3-hour shorter first stage (10 hours compared to 13.5) and multiparas experiencing 2 hours less of labor than those who were supine in labor (Table 4-3). The second stage was considerably shortened for both primiparas and multiparas in the squatting groups. Similar to the Golay study, findings were that squatting for delivery showed no increase in fetal complications at births, as measured by an Apgar score of less than 5 at birth.

The major difference in this study from the Golay findings is that these two authors, both obstetricians, found significantly greater "maternal injuries" in the squatting group: 38 cases, compared to 14 in the supine group. In their discussion, it is noted that all 46 primiparas in the supine groups were given "prophylactic episiotomies" and episiotomy was not included as "maternal injury." The authors further note:

> Initially for the first 22 primigravidae in the squatting group no episiotomies were given but with the high incidence of perineal trauma encountered, the remaining 20 primigravidae were

TABLE 4-3   Length of First and Second Stage in Squatting and Supine Positions

Variable	First Stage (in hours)	Second Stage (in mins)
Squatting primip (n = 42)	10.5	25
Supine primip (n = 46)	13.5	45
Squatting multip (n = 58)	6.0	16.5
Supine multip (n = 54)	8.0	30

Adapted from Allahbadia and Vaidya (1991). Table 3 from Squatting Position for Delivery as published in Journal of the Indian Medical Association Volume 91(1): 13–16. Used with permission.

given a prophylactic episiotomy at which moment they had to lie down in a supine position temporarily. *No support was given to the perineum at the time of delivery of the baby in the squatting position* [italics added by author].

Of the 38 recorded "maternal injuries" among the squatting group, 13 were "extension of episiotomy," with no comment being made that this complication perhaps resulted from the fact that an episiotomy was cut, rather than from the squat position. "First and second degree tears" were also counted as maternal complications, even though readers have no idea whether these required suturing or not. In their conclusions, these authors indicate ambulating in labor is useful, but they report that as an outcome of the study, they stopped delivery in the upright position until proper birth chairs can be acquired. There is no discussion of introducing routine support for the perineum at the time of birth as an option, nor of allowing the mother herself to decide what position she would prefer for delivery.

These two studies are discussed together to reveal how assumptions and biases can influence research. The first study included two nurse midwife-researchers who saw as positive outcomes the findings that there were significantly fewer and less severe perineal lacerations and fewer episiotomies in the squatting group. The physician-researchers in the second study saw lack of episiotomy, leading to any tear, as a negative finding. A later chapter discusses episiotomy as an intervention linked to breastfeeding, but for now it is important to note that substantial evidence points to upright postures making labor and delivery faster, and also that more upright postures are not linked to adverse outcomes in the fetus or newborn. Both of these findings would positively impact early initiation of breastfeeding in that the mother will be less tired and the newborn is in good health.

The newborn's well-being is an important component of early, effective breastfeeding. Two recent studies, one in Bulgaria with 36 women at term[10] and the other in Germany with 56 women in labor,[11] used a pulse oximeter to measure fetal oxygenation as it varied with different maternal position. Findings were that the supine position was least favorable for optimal oxygenation of the fetus.

Electronic Fetal Monitoring and Position for Labor

The use of routine electronic fetal monitoring (EFM) for monitoring normal labor has been questioned for over 20 years and researched from many perspectives. A full discussion of this research is beyond the scope of this chapter. *A Guide to Effective Care in Pregnancy and Childbirth,* based on Cochrane reviews, reports 12 randomized controlled clinical trials on EFM, representing over 58,000 laboring women and comparing EFM to routine intermittent auscultation with a fetoscope.[12] In all the studies, instrumental delivery and cesarean section rates were higher in the EFM groups, and the authors note that when there was not the added technology of fetal scalp pH sampling to assess true fetal distress, the cesarean section rates were "much" greater. The authors report no evidence that perinatal death rates or low Apgar scores were improved with EFM. There was evidence that neonatal seizures are fewer with "continuous EFM." The authors do note the disadvantages of limited mobility in the laboring woman who is undergoing EFM, and upright position and ambulation in normal labor are recommended. (See Figures 4-6 and 4-7.)

For the purposes of this chapter, perhaps the key points about EFM are:

- A woman undergoing EFM is confined to bed (unless there is capability for "walking telemetry" which is very expensive and uncommon).
- EFM conveys a clear message to a woman in labor, through the belts and leads and machinery, that she and her unborn baby are labor patients who must be monitored with noisy and often intimidating technology. Moving to and from the toilet or changing position in bed becomes a problem, requiring the assistance of a nurse.

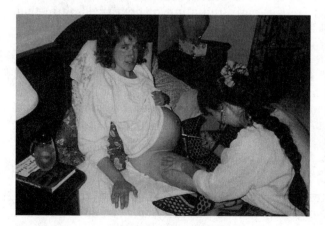

FIGURE 4-6 Here the midwife (who is also the continuous labor support companion) does intermittent auscultation of fetal heartbeat with a fetoscope, as Susan sits upright in bed. Hands-on fetal monitoring is cost-effective, as safe as EFM, and allows for a mother-friendly personal touch. *Photo used with permission, 1990.*

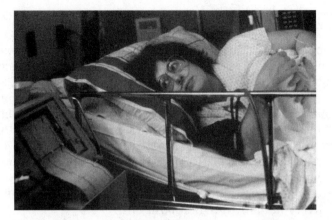

FIGURE 4-7   Routine electronic fetal monitoring has proved to be unnecessary for healthy mothers, restricts the mother to bed, and puts labor management decisions in the hands of obstetrical care providers who "interpret" how her labor is progressing by the machine. *Photo © Kip Kozlowski. Used with permission.*

- If there is "internal" monitoring, the fetal scalp must be lanced to allow the application of the monitor lead. This causes pain to the fetus and may have impact on the newborn's comfort in breastfeeding postpartum (see Chapter 7).
- There is a well-documented association between apparently false interpretations of fetal distress with EFM, which if not confirmed with additional fetal blood sampling, lead to a rush for instrumental or cesarean delivery. These interventions bring another cascade of interventions, which may impact breastfeeding (see Chapters 7 and 8).

The revised *Guidelines for Perinatal Care,* published in 2002 jointly by the American College of Obstetricians and Gynecologists (ACOG) and the American Academy of Pediatrics (AAP), has no discussion or recommendation on ambulation or positions in labor or delivery.[13] There is discussion of the use of "appropriate" EFM, with nothing that qualifies what is "appropriate." There is no mention of the disadvantage of EFM, as it requires confinement to bed. Given the 12 clinical trials discussed by the Cochrane database cited in the preceding paragraphs, the absence of a full discussion of the pros and cons of this intervention by ACOG and AAP is surprising.

Labor Position in Childbirth in Developing Countries

In Europe and Australia, early studies that laid the scientific basis for getting women in labor off their backs led to changes in practice. In the United States, in spite of the persisting ACOG and AAP guidelines discussed in the preceding section, maternity care providers, particularly midwives, do encourage ambulation and upright position. Many hospitals now have maternity beds with controls that can convert the bed into a modified birthing chair, and many have squat bars that allow the woman to more easily stay upright for pushing. Birth centers encourage delivery in the position of the woman's choice, and midwives in these settings are trained to be comfortable with delivery in many different positions.

Yet, despite changes made in Western countries, bed rest in labor and the supine and lithotomy positions for delivery continue to be common practices in developing countries worldwide. In the author's work over the last two decades in Central America, Anglophone Africa, Central Asia, Cambodia, and Indonesia, women in government maternity facilities are still put to bed in labor and are routinely flat on their backs for delivery, frequently with their legs in stirrups. Many hospital-based nurses, midwives, and doctors in developing countries have never seen a delivery with the mother upright or in the squat position. Refresher training can be an opportunity to introduce upright and squatting position delivery to these health care providers (Figure 4-8). It many be necessary to mentor the staff, who are used to having control over when and how the mother pushes, when to apply drapes, when to cut an episiotomy, and when to hand the newborn to the mother after delivery. A mother on her back in stirrups is not in a position of power in the birth relationship.

Traditional midwives* in many countries still use upright positions for delivery, but even these practices are changing. Training programs for traditional birth attendants often teach the use of a washable plastic sheet, generally included in "TBA birth kits." This is provided so the mother can lie down on a clean surface for the delivery. This "equipment" has discouraged what may have been an established cultural norm of the mother being upright in some settings.

---

*Traditional midwives are sometimes called traditional birth attendants or TBAs. They have learned midwifery from relatives or by experience rather than through formal academic training.

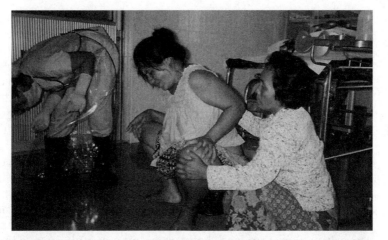

FIGURE 4-8   Midwife in Cambodia (at left) observes the "new" practice of squatting for the second stage of labor. The patient's mother was permitted into the delivery room to support her daughter. When the baby's head was visible, the delivery was completed on the delivery table. *Photo by Mary Kroeger (ACNM Life Savings Skills training, Cambodia, 2001).*

Conclusions

Given the lack of clinical research that links upright positions in labor and delivery directly to breastfeeding outcomes, one observational study is worth describing. Dr. Moyses Paciornik produced a powerful teaching video in 1979 based on his work in Southern Brazil.[14] Depicted are five mothers who were filmed in the squatting position in the second stage of labor, during delivery, and immediately postpartum. The hospital provided a special platform for squatting delivery with padded toweling on the floor, and all five mothers give birth to normal infants with very minimal involvement of an attendant.

Each mother, after regaining her composure for a few seconds from the intensity of the delivery, looks down, touches and strokes her infant, and then picks up and cuddles her baby. Some put the baby to breast. The mothers are the first to touch their newborns and there is no interference from staff (although it is assumed that they cut and clamped the umbilical cords). The environment is very peaceful. What is striking about this video is that the natural continuum of second stage of labor, delivery, and immediate bonding and breastfeeding is so evident. When using the video for training of hospital birth attendants in Central and Southeast Asia and

Africa there is often disbelief from doctors, midwives, and nurses alike with typical statements being "This is impossible!" or "Women in our country could never do this" or "Doesn't the perineum tear?" Many hospital birth attendants will need to learn (or relearn) about the positional advantage and implicit empowerment that can come to a mother who is not supine with her legs strapped into stirrups on a hard, narrow table at the time of delivery.

The French doctor Michael Odent was an important influence in reeducating the obstetrical world to the importance of birth in the "supported squat" position. While a practicing obstetrician, Odent openly advocated for the return to birthing in "quiet, dark, out of the way corners with a woman free to assume whatever position she chooses."[15] He discussed the anatomic and physiologic advantages of upright delivery and emphasized the absolute priority of mother and baby remaining a unit in a climate of warmth, intimacy, and with skin-to-skin contact. Initiation of breastfeeding is a natural extension of the delivery process for his patients. Odent has written extensively in the last two decades on the connection between labor, delivery, and breastfeeding.[15–17]

Summary Points for Protecting the Mother-Baby Continuum

- Evidence from randomized controlled clinical trials documents that an upright position during the second stage of labor leads to faster deliveries, fewer instrumental deliveries, less perceived pain, and fewer episiotomies.
- Women should be encouraged to use upright positions for labor and delivery, in so far as prolonged labor, instrumental deliveries, episiotomy, and need for pain medication are factors associated with breastfeeding difficulties.
- There is no evidence that continuous electronic fetal monitoring improves maternal or long-term newborn outcomes, and it generally requires that the mother remain in bed.

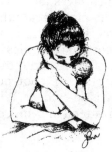

References

1. Ashford JI. 1986. *Mothers and Midwives: A History of Traditional Childbirth.* Booklet and slide set. Self-published and out of print. *www.jashford.com.*

2. DeLee JB. 1924. *Principles and Practice of Obstetrics,* 4th ed. Philadelphia and London: WB Saunders.

3. Caldeyro-Barcia, et al. 1960. Effect of position changes on the intensity and frequency of uterine contractions during labor. *Am J Obstet Gynecol,* 80:285.

4. Caldeyro-Barcia R. 1979. The influence of maternal position during second stage of labor. *Birth and Family Journal,* 6(1):31–42.

5. Bieniarz J, Maqueda E, Caldeyro-Barcia R. 1966. Compression of aorta by the uterus in late pregnancy. I. Variations between femoral and brachial artery pressure with changes from hypertensions to hypotension. *Am J Obstet Gynecol,* 95(6): 795–808.

6. Declercq ER, Sakala C, Corry MP, Applebaum S, Risher P. 2002. *Listening to Mothers: Report of the First National U.S. Survey of Women's Childbearing Experiences,* New York: Maternity Center Association, October 2002.

7. Gupta JK, Nikodem VC. 2001. Women's position during second stage of labour (Cochran review) In: The Cochran Library, Issue 3, 2001. Oxford: Update software.

8. Golay J, Vedam S, Sorger L. 1993. The squatting position for the second stage of labor: Effects on labor and on the maternal and fetal well-being. *Birth,* 20(2):73–78.

9. Allahbadia GN, Vaidya PR. 1991. Squatting position for delivery. *J Indian Med Assoc,* 91(1):13–15.

10. Nilolov A, Dimitrov A, Kovachev L. 2001. Influence of maternal position during delivery of fetal oxygen saturation [in Bulgarian]. *Akush Ginekol* (Sofia) 40(3):8–10.

11. Schmidt S, Sierra F, Hess C, et al. 2001. [Effect of modified labor position on oxygenation of the fetus-a pulse oximetry study—in German]. *Z Geburtshilfe Neonatal* 205(2):49–53.

12. Enkin M, Keirse M, Renfrew M, Neilson J. 2000. *A Guide to Effective Care in Pregnancy and Childbirth,* 3rd ed. Oxford: Oxford University Press.

13. Gilstrip LC, Oh W, Eds. 2002. *Guidelines for Perinatal Care,* 5th ed. Jointly published by the American College of Obstetrics and Gynecology and the American Academy of Pediatrics.

14. Paciornik M. 1979. *Birth in the Squatting Position.* Rev. version, 2001. Video. Sherman Oaks, CA: Academy Communications.

15. Odent M. 1984. *Birth Reborn.* New York: Pantheon Books.

16. Odent M. 1992. *The Nature of Birth and Breast-feeding.* Westport, CT: Bergan and Garvey.

17. Odent M. 1999. *The Scientification of Love.* London: Free Association Books Limited.

CHAPTER 5

ORAL FLUIDS, FOOD, AND IV HYDRATION IN LABOR AND BREASTFEEDING

"The odds of dying of aspiration in labor are less that that of being struck by lightning twice in one year."

Martha Sleutel and Susan S Golden, Registered Nurses, 1991

Left to their own instincts, women in labor will typically eat and drink lightly during early labor. As contractions intensify, they tend to take sips of liquids when offered, but otherwise take very little. This observation is based on the author's clinical practice during 27 years as a nurse and midwife in attendance at hundreds of deliveries in a multitude of cultures and settings. The observation is also corroborated in the literature.[1-3]

With the move to the hospital for delivery and the introduction in the 1940s of more general anesthesia used during labor such as ether, the protocol in the United States was to withhold any food and drink during labor to prevent any possibility of vomiting and subsequent aspiration pneumonia. As the use of general anesthesia for ordinary labor became less common, this practice of taking in nothing by mouth has continued, in spite of no compelling evidence that this practice was warranted.[4,5] Linked to this practice in many hospitals is the routine administration of intravenous (IV) fluids, often upon admission to the maternity ward in labor. Once a woman is attached to an IV line, her physical and psychological mobility are hampered and she truly becomes a "patient." Even in the best of circumstances with a portable IV pole, a woman loses the autonomy of freely taking any position in which she feels most comfortable and her fluid intake is monitored by a health provider rather than being driven by her own thirst (Figure 5-1).

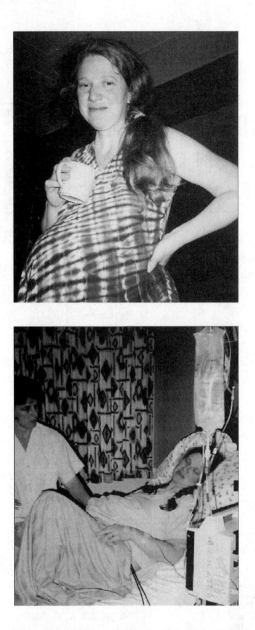

FIGURE 5-1 (Top) Susan in early labor at home drinking herbal tea with honey. Besides being free to eat and drink as she wants, she is also wearing her own clothing, walking, and staying upright during contractions. (Bottom) After admission to the hospital, Susan is in bed with an IV, hospital gown, and electronic fetal monitor in place. The atmosphere of self-determination is removed and she assumes the "patient" role. *Photos by John McNamer, British Columbia, 1989.*

Literature Reviews on Eating and Drinking in Labor

Literature reviews on the practice of withholding oral intake in labor abound,[1,4–8] and they all conclude, some more passionately than others, that there is no scientific justification for this lingering practice. One of the more recent reviews, done by two clinical nurse educators, categorized data under headings: historical review, effects of fasting on labor, research on maternal mortality/morbidity from aspiration, research on gastric emptying in labor, IV hydration in labor, and implication for nursing research.[5] These authors found that there is little research on how fasting versus allowing oral food and fluids in labor directly impacts labor, delivery, or the newborn. Their analysis of the cumulative data led them to conclude that there is no evidence that restricting oral intake in labor prevents gastric aspiration, nor is there evidence that there is risk in allowing them. Finally, they conclude that there is some evidence that substituting IV therapy for oral hydration may have unexpected negative outcomes for both mother and baby. Yet these authors report that most hospitals in the United States in 1999 continued to restrict oral intake to ice chips or sips of clear liquids only.

Labor as Vigorous Exercise

To meet the energy requirements during pregnancy, pregnant women in the United States are encouraged to eat at least an additional 200–300 kcal more per day.[9] Breastfeeding mothers are counseled to eat approximately 500–650 additional kcal per day during lactation, depending on their postpartum weight.[10] It is surprising, then, that for at least six decades women in maternity wards have been told they cannot eat or drink freely during labor, a time when their caloric needs are intensified.

Hazle, a nurse midwife, published one of the first literature reviews on hydration in labor in the mid 1980s when common practice in the United States was routine IV administration in labor.[6] This article gives an overview of how physiologic dehydration is monitored in labor and raises the question as to whether limiting oral intake and substituting IV therapy in labor is appropriate. Maternity nurses routinely monitor the urine of women in labor to check for ketones, and use their presence as a sign of dehydration. Ketones occur when carbohydrate stores are used up, and the author's discussion of dehydration in labor notes:

> In labor, this tendency [in pregnancy] towards ketosis is accentuated by increased muscular activity and by the starvation that

is usually imposed by limiting oral intake to ice chips. As carbohydrate stores are used up, keto-genesis is stimulated.

Hazle compares the work done by a woman's uterine muscle in labor to an athletic competition and suggests that rather than "starving" a woman in labor, it is better to have a "pregame meal" and additional oral fluids in early labor so that when a woman enters the active phase of labor—the real game—she is well nourished and hydrated. In active labor, the desire to eat and drink varies and a women should follow her body signals for satisfying thirst and hunger.

IV Therapy and the Mother and Newborn

Hazle's review also points out some harmful effects of IV therapy both on the mother and the newborn. There are risks of fluid overload in a mother who has an IV in place that is not closely monitored by maternity staff. She notes two studies whereby laboring women received far more IV fluids than had been ordered, as measured by the postpartum colloidal osmotic pressure; although they adjusted postpartum to this overload, some had received almost twice the amount of IV fluids ordered.[11,12] Most women can adjust to a moderate fluid imbalance unless they have an underlying cardiopulmonary disease, in which case fluid overload could have serious health consequences.

Examples are cited of excessive water loads in laboring women having an impact on their infants, who had problems with hypoglycemia (low blood sugar), hyponatremia (low sodium), and jaundice.[13-14] A more recent review of the literature on eating and drinking in labor corroborates these findings of electrolyte imbalances in newborns of mothers who received IV therapy.[1]

What impact do these "rebound" electrolyte imbalances have on the newborn? Among the more compelling studies cited in the 1993 review is one done by Singhi[15] and associates in Jamaica. They studied term infants of mothers who received intravenous glucose therapy during spontaneous labor and oxytocin induced labor. They reported that 5% glucose infusions in labor were associated with increases in neonatal hyponatremia and transient tachypnea (rapid breathing). In addition, the newborns in the hyponatremic group developed jaundice (54%) more often, compared to the normo-natremic infants (21%). Since clinical management of neonatal jaundice involves infants who may be separated for phototherapy and who are frequently lethargic, an association with increased breastfeeding difficulties could exist.[16,17]

A later randomized controlled study by Singhi examined the influence of IV therapy in laboring mothers and newborn glucose levels in 45 infants of healthy mothers with normal deliveries.[18] Twenty-three of the infants (study group) were of mothers who received 5% or 10% dextrose IV in labor either for hydration or for oxytocin induction, and 22 were infants of mothers with no IVs (controls). At delivery, both groups of infants were similar with respect to maternal and prenatal variables, APGAR scores, and birth weight. Blood glucose levels in the infants measured at one and two hours postpartum showed that study infants were three times more likely to be hypoglycemic (have low blood sugar as defined as 2.2 mm/l or less). Neurobehavioral evaluation using the Early Neonatal Neurobehavioral Scale (ENNS) was administered at one and two hours of age on all infants. The hypoglycemic infants had a significantly lower average score on muscle tone and delayed habituation to various stimuli (Moro reflex extinction and response to pin prick and light). Infants showed "significant lowering of muscle tone, and delayed habituation to various stimuli at one to two hours of age." There was no statistical difference between suck and root reflex in either group. There is no information about early contact between mothers and newborns nor whether they breastfed.

Fluid Overload and Possible Effects on Breastfeeding

Not surprisingly, no studies were found directly linking breastfeeding outcomes to hydration in labor (by any mode, whether oral or IV). However, hyponatremia in infants is associated with convulsions, respiratory distress, feeding difficulties, and excess water loss after birth.[15,18] Hypoglycemic infants are often separated from their mothers for serial blood tests and observation and if the imbalance persists, these infants may become lethargic, jittery, or may have convulsions.[19] The evidence from the studies reviewed suggests that inappropriate use of intravenous therapy in labor can lead to electrolyte imbalance in the newborn. A newborn blood sample, which is usually taken by puncturing the infant's heel with a lancet, causing pain and crying, may show hypoglycemia while the newborn is asymptomatic. Hypoglycemia is a common reason for early supplementation with glucose water or formula and often leads to separation of mother and baby in the early postpartum period when bonding and breastfeeding are being established. If there is early separation of the mother-baby dyad, there are two highly significant risks for disruption of breastfeeding: non-timely initiation of breastfeeding and offering of fluids other than colostrum[20,21] (also see Chapter 10 on skin-to-skin contact).

Fluid overload has known and unknown consequences to the infant and the process of lactogenesis (onset of lactation). Lactation consultants have reported severe cases of breast, nipple, and areolar edema on the second or third postpartum day that seem to be correlated with IV fluid hydration and/or induction of labor. Mechanically, edema in the breast causes the infant to have a difficult time latching on, and may trigger poor oral-motor behavior causing nipple pain and poor milk transfer. The mother may become reluctant to put her baby to breast because of breast pain. Theoretically, fluid overload could have an effect on the process of lactogenesis. Maternal serum provides many of the components that are fashioned into milk components by the lactocytes (secretory mammary epithelial cells) in the mammary gland.[22] In animal studies, low serum albumin delays the onset of lactogenesis II (copious milk production).

It is known that oxytocin acts as an antidiuretic and oxytocin augmentation and induction in labor can cause fluid retention in the mother.[23] Humenick and Hill have studied postpartum breast engorgement and have identified several factors, including mode of delivery, pariety, and previous experience with breastfeeding as factors contributing to this condition.[24-25] Neither intravenous therapy nor oxytocin infusion in labor were examined as variables in their studies. It would be interesting for such a study to be done to determine if there is a relationship to later development. There is also evidence that intravenous therapy in labor contributes to newborns who may be "water logged." Dahlenburg reported that for babies whose mothers had intravenous fluids, percentage weight loss was 6.17 +/− 3.36 (SD) percent as opposed to 4.07 (+/−2.20 (SD) percent for those whose mothers had only oral fluids (P < 0.01).[26] Excessive infant weight loss in the early neonatal period is often a reason for aggressive supplementation.

Oral Intake and Labor Outcomes

Two randomized controlled trials have examined different aspects of oral intake in labor. One done in the United Kingdom examined

48 women who were given a "light" diet in labor compared to a control group of 46 women who were permitted only water.[27] The outcomes measured included: 1) alteration in the maternal metabolic profile, 2) differences in outcome of labor, and 3) increase in gastric volumes (as a theoretical risk for pulmonary aspiration). Results showed that there was no difference between the two groups in duration of labor, oxytocin requirements, or mode of delivery. Nor were there differences in the newborns' Apgar scores or umbilical arterial or venous blood samples. They did find that eating in labor prevented ketosis (a sign of inadequate caloric intake). Although development of ketosis in this study was not linked to adverse effects on labor in either group, it is documented that severe ketosis has been associated with prolonged labor.[28] A further finding was that the eating group had a significantly greater residual gastric volume, but no clinical significance was attributed to this finding.

Another randomized controlled double-blinded trial, conducted in the Netherlands, researched whether oral glucose intake could have a detrimental impact on fetal metabolic acidosis as has been reported in instances of IV glucose administration.[29] The study randomized 100 nulliparas (first-time mothers) into two groups. One group received 200 ml of a 25-gram glucose solution at 8–10 centimeters dilation and the other group received a placebo drink at the same stage of labor. Both subjects and care providers were blind as to what each mother received. Findings were that the fetal arterial blood pH was similar in both groups and was physiologically within normal limits. The authors conclude that oral carbohydrate intake during late labor seems safe in regards to fetal metabolic status. These studies, along with the findings from the Sleutel, et al. literature review, argue against "starving" a woman in labor and argue for encouraging a mother to choose light food and drink to her own taste in order to prevent ketosis.

Psychological Effects of Withholding Oral Intake and of IVs

Advocates for keeping birth normal have questioned the use of routine IVs for normal healthy labor, given the restriction on movement and pain associated with maternal IV therapy.[30] Two of these authors have also examined the literature reviewing historical practices and cross-cultural practices on oral intake in labor.[31] In a separate article in the same journal they reviewed the literature that advocated prohibition of oral intake in labor, and they advocate a much closer look at the psychological effects of this practice in hospitals as it compares to unrestricted feeding in the homebirth setting. They conclude that this continued practice in hospitals reflects "culture lag" within obstetrics. Around the same time, a childbirth educator studied "stressful" childbirth events in the United States among new mothers and reported that 27% of the mothers interviewed rated restriction of food in labor as moderately to most stressful and 57% found restriction of fluids to be moderately to most stressful.[32] Also, 58% of mothers in this survey reported IV therapy in labor as "moderately or most stressful."

Even in a "low-intervention" model of care, the attitudes of the care providers may influence the method by which a laboring mother is hydrated. One small qualitative study using in-depth interviews of four registered nurses and five certified nurse midwives who worked together in a birth center setting, found that nurses are more likely to offer IVs than midwives.[8] The discussion attributes this to the differing roles the two professions played in care provision. The midwives were more likely to "satisfy client preference and resort to IVs only when all other options ran out." All of the nurses interviewed had previously worked in conventional hospital settings where IV therapy had been routine, and they "expressed more concern over the timing and placement of the IV [which was their responsibility] within their overall workload" and prior to an emergency situation.

A prospective study published in the Netherlands in 2001 looked at a randomly selected group of midwives and obstetricians from the whole country as to what advice they gave to their patents regarding eating and drinking in labor.[33] Nulliparous mothers (N = 211) were questioned after delivery as to: 1) whether they had been advised to take food and drink in labor, 2) if they had followed the advice, and 3) what they had actually taken. After adjusting for possible confounding factors, it was seen that mothers who had been given advice to take food and drink took the advice, and 75% of these women took solid food. After further adjusting for prognostic factors, the researchers found that the incidence of instrumental deliveries due to a non-progressing second stage of labor was significantly lower: 10 (12.5%) of the women who had caloric intake versus 32 (24%) of the women who had not (p = 0.04). Chapter 7 discusses evidence suggesting that instrumental delivery is associated with greater difficulties in establishing breastfeeding, and thus here we must consider the indirect impact of withholding calories by mouth during labor, leading to assisted delivery, and thus affecting breastfeeding.

Hydration in Labor in Developing Countries and Resource-Poor Settings

The issue of hydration and nutrition in labor is still problematic in many developing countries where forbidding oral intake in labor is still common practice. Where resources are scarce and IV fluids are not widely available for any but the most serious emergencies, this practice means that women labor for hours, even in hot, tropical climates, without even water to drink. With training and dissemination of new information, this practice is gradually changing. In Cambodia, the head midwife in a busy provincial maternity hospital "broke the long-standing rules" and allowed family members of women admitted in labor to bring bottled water, sweetened teas, and soft drinks (see Figure 5-2). She agreed to this as part of a new "Life Savings Skills" package that was being introduced through training to the maternity staff midwives. She observed at the end of the first four weeks of training that of all the "new" ideas that had been introduced through the training, offering fluids to the mothers in labor had been the most

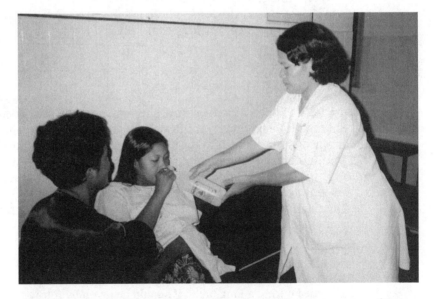

FIGURE 5-2　Staff midwife in Cambodia offers bottled water to a mother in active labor as one of the new techniques in the "Life Savings Skills" training program with the Ministry of Health. *Photo by M. Kroeger, ACNM LSS Training, Phnom Penh, 2001.*

important change. She said that she had observed happier mothers and that when she had compiled her monthly data she had noted faster labors and better newborn Apgar scores.[34]

The WHO/IMPAC guide for midwives and doctors in developing country settings recommends the following: "Encourage the woman to eat and drink as she wishes. If the woman has visible severe wasting or tires easily during labor, make sure she is fed. Nutritious liquid drinks are important, even in late labor."[35] In a later section, where prolonged labor is discussed, the recommendation states: "If acetone (ketones) is present in the woman's urine, suspect poor nutrition and give dextrose IV."

When IVs are used, 5% dextrose or glucose is still the IV fluid most commonly available in resource-poor settings for women in labor. Frequently there are no alternatives. Unless there is a clear medical indication for IV fluid replacement, it is more prudent to encourage oral intake of locally available and acceptable liquids with a caloric content, including juices, teas with sugar, coconut water, fruit smoothies, and even carbonated soft drinks. In a healthy pregnancy, the mother's circulatory and renal system, along with the placenta, are better equipped to regulate the fluids, electrolytes, and glucose absorbed by her digestive tract than direct glucose intravenous infusions, which reach the baby far more rapidly and often in concentrations that may be detrimental.

Culture Lag

Culture lag has been described as a phenomenon wherein a "culturally patterned behavior continues to be practiced long after the major reasons for doing so have disappeared."[31] These authors used this terminology for the practice of fasting in labor. Culture lag is reflected in the 2002 *Guidelines for Perinatal Care*, jointly published by the American College of Obstetrics and Gynecology (ACOG) and the American Academy of Pediatrics (AAP). In the section on normal labor management, the guidelines read:

> Patients in active labor should avoid oral ingestion of anything except sips of clear liquids, occasional ice chips, or preparations for moistening the mouth and lips. When significant hydration is needed during a long labor, it should be given by intravenous infusion.[36]

These guidelines are published for obstetrics and pediatric care in the United States, and the Introduction states "it is encouraging to note that there is increasing use of single and muticenter trials to assess the efficacy and safety of therapeutic interventions in maternal and fetal medicine and neonatology." Yet this policy on labor hydration disregards the existing evidence (see Box 5-1). Is this simply "culture lag" or is it more systematic? Reflecting back on Michel Odent's discussion of approaches to research (covered in Chapter 2), it seems closer to "cul-de-sac" research in which "findings are shunned by the medical community and the media."[38]

In contrast, Enkin et al., the counterpart guide used in the United Kingdom discusses the lack of evidence for and disadvantages of fasting in labor, stating that "enforced fasting may also lead to poor progress in labor, the diagnosis of dystocia, and a cascade of interventions, culminating in a cesarean section." These authors recommend as a reasonable alternative to fasting: "a low residue, low-fat diet with the aim of providing palatable, attractive, small meals at frequent intervals." They continue, "the effects of routine IV therapy should be weighed against the alternative option of allowing a women to eat and drink as they desire."[39]

Box 5-1   "Culture Lag" is Still Lagging

The recent *Listening to Mothers* survey of childbearing experiences in the United States among 1583 women who responded to telephone interviews or electronic mail surveys reported that 86% of respondants had IV therapy in labor. Only one in three women (34%) reported that they had been permitted to drink anything, and one in eight had been permitted food of any kind (13%). When the respondents who ended up with cesarean sections were eliminated from the data set, still only 35% of woman having vaginal births drank in labor and only 14% took solid foods.[37]

Conclusions

Where does this leave breastfeeding outcomes? No studies were found that looked at the method of labor hydration—whether with IV, fasting, or allowing oral intake—and tested the impact on mothers' physiologic readiness to initiate breastfeeding. Studies do document women's verbalized stress experiences with IVs and enforced fasting. Certainly what is known about athletic performance as well as simple logic suggests that a well-hydrated and nourished mother is in the best condition to deliver normally and to hold and bond with her newborn and initiate breastfeeding.

Summary Points for Protecting the Mother-Baby Continuum

- There is evidence that withholding food and drink in labor is an outdated and unjustifiable practice that does not improve birth outcomes.
- There is evidence that some commonly used IV solutions can lead to electrolyte imbalances, jaundice, and other problems in the newborn, requiring special treatment that could involve separation from the mother and thus impact early breastfeeding.
- Evidence suggests that withholding oral intake and instituting IV therapy is perceived by mothers as painful, stressful, and restrictive of movement in labor, and thus can lead to prolonged labor and other interventions that could impact early breastfeeding.

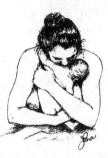

References

1. Ludka LM and Roberts CC. 1993. Eating and drinking in labor: A literature review. *J Nurse Midwifery* 38(4):199–201.
2. O'Reilly SA, Perrone-Hoyer PJP, Walsh E. 1993. Low-risk mothers: Oral intake and emesis in labor. *J Nurse Midwifery* 38(4):199–207.
3. Rooks JP, Weatherby NL, Ernst EKM. 1992. The national birth center study. Part II: Intrapartum and immediate postpartum and neonatal care. *J Nurse Midwifery* 37(5):301–330.
4. Elkington KW. 1991. At the waters edge where obstetrics and anesthesia meet. *Obstet Gynecol* 77(2):304–308.
5. Sleutel M and Golden SS. 1999. Fasting in labor: Relic or requirement. *JOGNN* 28(5):507–512.
6. Hazle NR. 1986. Hydration in labor: Is routine intravenous hydration necessary? *J Nurse Midwifery* 31(4):171–176.

7. Broach J and Newton N.1988. Food and beverages in labor. Part II: the effects of cessation of oral intake during labor. *Birth* 15(2):88–92.

8. Sommer PA, Norr K, Roberts J. 2000. Clinical decision-making regarding intravenous hydration in normal labor in a birth center setting. *J Midwife Womens Health* 45(2):114–121.

9. Institute of Medicine. 1990. *Nutrition During Pregnancy.* Washington, DC: National Academy of Sciences.

10. Dewey KG. 1997. Energy and protein requirements during lactation. *Annual Review of Nutrition* 17:19–36.

11. Cotton DB, et al. 1984. Intrapartum to postpartum changes in colloidal osmotic pressure. *Am J Obstet Gynecol* 142(2):174–176.

12. Gonik B, Cotton DB. 1984. Peripartum colloid osmotic pressure changes: Influence of intravenous hydration. *Am J Obstet Gynecol* 150(1):99–100.

13. Jawalekar S, Marx GF. 1980. Effect of IV fluids on maternal and fetal blood glucose. *Anesthesiology* 53(3):311S.

14. Lucas A, Adrain TE, Aynsley-Green A. 1980. Iatrogenic hyperinsulinism at birth. *Lancet* 1(8160):144–145.

15. Singhi S, Chookang E, Hall J, et al. 1985. Iatrogenic neonatal and maternal hyponatremia following oxytocin and aqueous glucose infusion during labor. *Br J Gynecol* 92:356–363.

16. Royal College of Midwives. 1991. *Successful Breastfeeding.* 2nd ed. Churchill Livingston, UK: Royal College of Midwives

17. Savage King F. 1992. *Helping Mothers to Breastfeed.* Rev. ed. Nairobi, Kenya: African Medical Research Foundation.

18. Singhi S. 1988. Effect of maternal intrapartum glucose therapy on neonatal blood glucose levels and neurobehavioral status of hypoglycemia term newborn infants. *J Perinat Med* 16:217–224.

19. Biancuzzo LM. 1999. *Breastfeeding the Newborn.* St. Louis: C V Mosby.

20. DiGirolamo AM, Grummer-Strawn LM, Fein S. 2001. Maternity care practices: Implications for breastfeeding. *Birth* 28(2):94–100.

21. Hill P, Humenick S, Breenon M, Wooley D. 1997. Does early supplementation affect long-term breastfeeding? *Clinical Pediatrics* 36:345–350.

22. Hartmann PE, Mitoulis LR, Kent J, et al. New insights into breast physiology and breast expression. Presentation at the International Lactation Consultant Association, 2002; based on research conducted at the University of Western Australia, 1990–2002.

23. Chou CL, DiGiovanni SR, Mejia R, et al. 1995. Oxytocin as a antidiuretic hormoneI. Concentration dependence of action. *Am J Physiol* 269 (1 Pt 2) 78–85.

24. Humenick SS, Hill PD, Anderson MA. 1984. Breast engorgement: patterns and selected Outcomes. *J Hum Lact* 10(2):87–93.

25. Hill PD and Humenick SS. 1984. The occurrence of breast engorgement. *J Hum Lact* 10(2):79–86.
26. Dahlenburg GW, Burnell RH, Braybrook R. 1980. The relationship between cord serum sodium levels in newborn infants and maternal intravenous therapy during labor. *Br J of Obstet Gynaecol.* 87:519-522.
27. Scrutton MJ, Metcalfe GA, Lowry C, et al. 1999. Eating in labor. A randomized controlled trial assessing the risks and benefits. *Anesthesia* 54(4):329–334.
28. Dumoulin JG and Foulke JEB. 1984. Ketonurea during labor. *Br Obstet Gynaecol* 91:97–98.
29. Scheepers HC, Thans MC, deJong PA, et al. 2002. The effects of oral carbohydrate administration on fetal acid base balance. *J Perinat Med* 30(5):400–404.
30. Newton N, Newton M, Broach J. 1988. Psychologic, nutritional, and technologic aspects of intravenous infusion during labor. *Birth.* 15(2):67–72.
31. Broach J and Newton N.1988a. Food and beverages in labor. Part I: Cross-cultural and historical practices. *Birth* 15(2):81–85.
32. Simkin P. 1986. Stress, pain, and catacholamines in labor. Part 2: Stress associated with childbirth events: A pilot survey of new mothers. *Birth* 33(4):234–240.
33. Scheepers HCJ, Thans MCJ, deJong P, et al. 2001. Eating and drinking in labor: The influence of caregiver advice on women's behavior. *Birth* 28(2):119–123.
34. Ma Setha.1999. Personal communication with Chief Maternity Unit, Battambang Hospital, Cambodia.
35. WHO, UNFPA, UNICEF, World Bank. 2000. Managing complications in Pregnancy and Childbirth: A guide for midwives and doctors. World Health Organization. Department of Reproductive Health and Research. WHO/RHR/00.7.
36. Gilstrip LC, Oh W, Eds. 2002. Guidelines for Perinatal care. 5th ed. Jointly published by the American College of Obstetrics and gynecology and the American Academy of Pediatrics.
37. Declercq ER, Sakala C, Corry MP, et al. 2002. *Listening to Mothers: Report of the First National U.S. Survey of Women's Childbearing Experiences.* New York: Maternity Center Association. October 2002. *www.maternity.org/listeningtomothers/ results.html.*
38. Odent M. 2000. Between circular and cul-de-sac epidemiology. *Lancet* 355(9212):1371.
39. Enkin M, Keirse M, Renfrew M, et al. 2000. *A Guide to Effective Care in Pregnancy and Childbirth.* 3rd ed. Oxford: Oxford University Press.

CHAPTER 6

LABOR PAIN MEDICATION AND BREASTFEEDING

"In labor I remember when my own endorphins kicked in...the pains were hard but in between them I was really flying high and I knew I could do it."

Adrianne Lyons Harrington, new mother, 2002

Background

It is not well understood why some women tolerate labor pain so much better than others. Common sense suggests that cultural expectations play a big role in setting a woman's attitude and expectations as she enters the childbirth experience. If a first-time mother expects that birth is dreadful and painful, if she has had no previous experience with unmedicated birth within her family, or if she has had no childbirth education on the normal progress of labor and ways to cope with its growing intensity, then she will likely ask for labor pain medicine if it is offered to her. In the United States in the 1930s, feminists and suffragist leaders heard about and demanded the miracle drug "twilight sleep," which was being used in childbirth in Europe.[1] This movement was successful and was embraced by obstetrics and during the first 50 years of the twentieth century, a wide variety of labor pain medicines were used, including spinal blocks of various types, inhalation gases, injectable opioids, and barbiturates. Twilight sleep is "a strange combination of sub-therapeutic doses of morphine and scopolamine designed to relieve some labor pain and render women amnesic for the rest of their labor."[2] However, twilight sleep was among the medications that became associated with severe respiratory depression in the newborn, and eventually it fell out of use. Were the same feminists who demanded the accessibility of twilight sleep in the early 1900s subsequently informed about and equally empowered to refuse its use once they knew it could have profound negative impact on the baby? This question is at the core of the discussion in this chapter, as there is a persistent failure on the part of both obstetrics and pediatrics to disclose to pregnant women the full range of possible side effects of labor pain medications.

Athletes are familiar with the phenomenon of "jogger's high," in which the human brain's hormonal response to extended physical stress releases endogenous opiates into the bloodstream. It is not as clear how this works in labor and birth, though it is reported that large concentrations of endorphins are secreted in labor.[3] Endorphins appear to help to reduce perception of uterine pain, provide a sense of well-being, and may have an amnesic effect. In an unmedicated labor in which a woman has good social support and feels safe and secure, birth attendants often observe that she becomes increasingly introverted with a dreamy, trancelike look. If she avoids other pain medicines, which can block the endorphins, she copes well, even during the hardest and strongest pains of the late first stage.[4] Andrea Robertson, a leading Australian childbirth educator, included a discussion of endogenous endorphins in all of her childbirth education classes and explained to mothers the antagonistic effect adrenaline has on this natural progress of labor.[5] With poor pain control and increased fear and anxiety, adrenaline works as an antagonist to oxytocin, weakens uterine contractions, prolongs labor, and may set the stage for IV oxytocin augmentation, medical pain relief, possible restriction to bed, electronic monitoring, and the possibility that an instrumental delivery or cesarean section will be performed. A surgical delivery deprives a woman of the empowering event of events of her life: pushing out her own baby while fully awake and in control, taking that baby immediately into her arms, and initiating the first breastfeed without interference. The other side of this partnership in childbirth is the baby and this chapter also examines the impact of labor pain medication on the newborn.

Literature Review on Childbirth Medication and Breastfeeding

The literature on analgesia and anesthesia during childbirth is vast and conflicting, but the preponderance of the evidence suggests that many routine labor medications can negatively impact the normalcy of labor and set in motion the cascade of interventions that can influence both the mother's physical well-being, alertness, and self-esteem and the newborn's readiness to see, smell, nuzzle, root, and attach on the mother's breast.

A classic study was done over 40 years ago by the renowned pediatrician T.B. Brazelton in a large urban hospital in the United States.[6] In this hospital, the routines did not facilitate breastfeeding, and infants were brought to their mothers to feed once in the first 24 hours after birth, twice in the second 24 hours, and so on. The anesthetics available included spinal, saddle blocks, pudendal blocks, and inhalants such as ether and nitrous oxide, and mothers who were given regional anesthesia were premedicated with scopolamine and barbiturates. Brazelton observed and measured a variety of newborn responses and also asked the mothers to evaluate their infants' alertness, attachment skill, and feeding duration at feeds over six days postpartum. He found that the extent of "relative central nervous system" disorganization or depression was positively correlated with the type, amount, and timing of medication given to the mother. Infants of mothers who had been minimally premedicated with scopolamine and barbiturates were rated as feeding well by 36–48 hours postpartum, whereas the infants of mothers heavily premedicated weren't feeding at the same rates until five to six days postpartum.

This sentinel study laid the basis for further investigation of the use of narcotic and barbiturate medications in labor and delivery. In 1973, Brazelton introduced his Neonatal Behavioral Assessment Scale (BNBAS) to assist researchers and clinicians in assessing early newborn psychophysiologic behavior.[7] This scale forms the basis of much of the research on newborn sleep/awake states and newborn ability to "self-organize." Later tools were developed that more closely allow assessment of newborn feeding behavior (see Box 6-1).

Box 6-1   Infant Clinical, Behavioral, Neurobehavioral, and Breastfeeding Assessment Tools

- The APGAR score, developed in 1952 by Virginia Apgar, provides a simple scoring system for evaluating the clinical status of a newborn at birth. The score ranges from 0 to 10; the more vigorous the infant the higher the score. The scoring is done at one minute and five minutes after delivery, and at again at ten minutes if the first two scores were low. Five gross essential parameters of newborn well-being at birth are measured, with each parameter receiving 0-2 points: heart rate, respiratory rate, muscle tone, reflex irritability, and color.[8]
- **The Brazelton Neonatal Behavior Assessment Scale (BNBAS)** served as the basis for earlier psychophysiologic assessment of newborn behavior after labor medication.[7] This tool, still used widely today, evaluates many aspects of the newborn's behavior, including states of consciousness (levels of sleep, levels of awake or alertness, and crying) reflexes, physiological responses to certain stresses, irritability/consolability, and a number of social interactive behaviors.
- **The Early Neonatal Neurobehavioral Scale (ENNS)**, developed by John W. Scanlon, is a more comprehensive neurobehavioral examination tool that includes APGAR scores, states of alertness and sleep, responses to numerous stimuli, and in regards to breastfeeding, assesses rooting and sucking reflexes.[9] This tool does not directly assess breastfeeding behavior.
- **The Infant Breastfeeding Assessment Tool (IBFAT)**, developed by M. Kay Matthews, has proved to be a valid instrument for assessing newborn breastfeeding readiness and success.[10] The IBFAT consists of a short questionnaire with six items. Two items are assessed qualitatively; one relates to the infant's alertness just before a feeding and the other relates to the mother's satisfaction with the feed. Four items rate specific breastfeeding behaviors: readiness to feed, rooting, latching, and sucking pattern. Each of these specific breastfeeding behaviors is rated from 0-3 points. A per-

fect IBFAT score is 12 and a 10–12 rating is counted as "effective" breastfeeding readiness.

- **The Via Christi Breastfeeding Assessment Tool** is a tool developed by Jan Riordan that specifically scores early breastfeeding behaviors and is intended to identify mothers and babies who will require close postpartum follow-up.[11] A full description of the tool, which is not referenced further in this book, can be found in the La Leche League International Lactation Consultant Series Two, Unit 4.[12]

Meperidine Effects on the Infant Central Nervous System

There are numerous studies from the 1980s implicating the use of the narcotic analgesic meperidine in labor (commercial names Demerol, Pethidine) as having a central nervous system depressive impact on newborns.[13–15] In spite of the findings of these studies, meperidine continued to be used as a labor analgesia worldwide. More recent studies have established additional newborn effects including impact on breastfeeding outcomes and these will be discussed.

The Righard and Alade (1990)[16] study from Sweden is well known to breastfeeding advocates because of the teaching video that was subsequently produced showing the newborn behaviors reported in the article.[17] This prospective observational study had two groups of mother-baby pairs. In one group (n = 38), the baby was left with the mother uninterrupted for an hour, or until they initiated breastfeeding. The other group of babies (n = 34) was removed at 20 minutes post delivery for bathing and weighing and then returned to the mother. There were babies in both groups from medicated and unmedicated labors. Findings were that of those infants whose mothers had received pethidine in labor (40 of 72 or 56%), 25 were too sedated to suck at all, 7 sucked in a disorganized manner and 8 sucked correctly. The statistical significance in these findings was high, and authors conclude that pethidine in labor is a highly significant deterrent to successful initiation of breastfeeding. Their discussion reports that the half-life of pethidine is 3–4.5 hours in the mother and as long as 13–23 hours in the newborn, with some of the metabolites remaining in the newborn's system even longer. This accounts for the central nervous system depression in these babies.

Another Swedish group studied the effects of pethidine for labor pain relief on newborn feeding behavior in a hospital where a common routine was to offer a relatively high dose (100 mg) of pethidine in labor.[18] In this quasi-experimental study, 44 mothers were observed immediately after birth in much the same manner as the Righard methodology. In this study the observer of the feeding behavior was blinded as to whether or not the mother had received pethidine in labor, making the likelihood of bias less than in the earlier study. Very specific breastfeeding behaviors were recorded during observations, including fist clenching, hand-to-mouth movements, rooting, sucking, and actual latching on. Of the 44 mothers, 18 received pethidine. Rooting and sucking movement and latch on were significantly delayed in the pethidine-exposed infants, but most eventually suckled. An interesting conclusion of the authors is that pethidine exposed infants should stay longer with their mothers to enable the infant to latch on. No recommendations are made that pethidine should be avoided as a labor medication and that alternative pain relief measures be used.

In England, a secondary analysis of a larger data set from the National Birthday Trust Fund survey tested the hypothesis that breastfeeding is inversely related to the amount of medical intervention in labor and delivery, and that some procedures have an impact on feeding.[19] A randomly chosen subset of 1149 of all mothers who had delivered in a certain week in 1990 responded to a postal questionnaire sent to their homes postpartum. There were questions about pain relief, health provider care, and experience with the birth, motherhood, and infant feeding. Results showed that there was significant difference in exclusive breastfeeding at six weeks in the non-pethidine group (45%) as compared to those who had received pethidine in labor (38%). Significantly more women were still breastfeeding at six weeks if they had had a vaginal delivery rather than an assisted or surgical delivery. The additional variable of prolonged second stage of labor also had a negative impact on breastfeeding at six weeks.

In the United States, the use of injected or IV Demerol and morphine was common for labor pain relief up until the early 1980s. It is likely that the combination of both the clinical concern over respiratory depression in the neonate and the growing consumer demand for awake and aware mothers and babies accounts for the drop in their use. Given the evidence that these narcotics have an impact on the neonatal central nervous system (CNS) and thus on early breastfeeding, it is surprising that Demerol (in Europe, Pethidine) continues to be used widely in much of Europe and the developing world. The WHO *Guide for Midwives and Doctors*, which is meant to provide guidelines for developing country settings, advocates the use of labor pain relief measures other than pharmacological methods, but states that "if necessary pethidine (up to 100 mg) or morphine can be given."[20] Bricker and Lavender's[21] extensive, systematic, and rigorous literature review on parenteral opioids for labor, presented at the 2001 symposium on The Nature and Management of Labor Pain, documents the early neonatal effects of meperidine and other opioids and calls for additional randomized controlled trials. Yet they also conclude that within this category of drug, meperidine is the drug of choice, stating: "Currently, intramuscular pethidine has the virtue of familiarity and low cost. Although there are considerable doubts about its effectiveness for maternal pain relief and concerns about its potential maternal, fetal, and newborn side effects." It seems that convenience and cost are more important than safety.

Newer, "Safer" Labor Drugs

By the 1970s, other Demerol-like medicines took the place of meperidine in the United States. Claims were that these synthetic narcotics have the advantages of fewer side effects (nausea and vomiting being the most common) for the mother, and shorter half-life, and thus more rapid placental clearing, before delivery. A Canadian midwife-researcher investigated breastfeeding behavior in 38 healthy term babies, based on the labor medication profile of the mothers.[10] A convenience sample of 20 mothers was used in the medicated group and 18 in the unmedicated control group. The standard labor analgesic given in the institution where the study occurred was alphaprodine (Nisentil), given either intramuscularly or IV.

This investigator developed an infant feeding scoring tool (IBFAT) for this research and was also using this research to validate the tool's effectiveness (see Box 6-1). The tool consists of a short questionnaire with six items. One item relates to the infant's alertness just before a feeding. This item is rated subjectively rather than given a numeric weight. This is also true of the sixth item, which relates to the mother's satisfaction with the feed. Items 2–5 relate specifically to the infant's feeding behavior (readiness to feed, rooting, latching sucking pattern), and these are scored numerically from 0–3 points, with a perfect score being 12. Results showed a significant difference in establishing breastfeeding between the babies whose mothers received alphaprodine between 1–3 hours before delivery compared to the control group, with the medicated mothers establishing breastfeeding on the average 21.2 hours after delivery versus 10.8 hours in the control group. A similar difference was not found if the medication had been given 1 hour or less prior to delivery. There are several scientific problems with this study, including lack of previous tool validation and self-scoring by the investigator. Nevertheless, the findings suggest that more research is warranted and that the effect of this medication needs to be considered for its impact on timely establishment of breastfeeding.

Two other commonly used analgesics for labor pain, butorphanol (Stadol) and nalbuphine (Nubain), were investigated by using the same IBFAT scoring tool.[22] A convenience sample of 120 breastfeeding mothers of first or second parity, who had just delivered healthy term singleton babies, was utilized. Mothers were grouped based on type of labor medication, and mothers of 48 newborns fit the study criteria for these medications. Effective breastfeeding was determined by scores of 10–12 on the IBFAT and time of initiation of breastfeeding was noted, "early" being <1 hour and "late" being >1 hour. Dose and timing of medications were included as variables. Findings were significant, with the mean hours for establishment of effective breastfeeding being 6.4 hours in the group that had initiated breastfeeding at less than 1 hour after birth and who had been unmedicated or medicated just prior to delivery. This is compared to mothers who also initiated breastfeeding at less than one hour of birth, but who had been medicated at an interval greater than one hour before delivery. This group established effective breastfeeding at a mean of 50.3 hours (see Table 6-1). The average time for establishment of effective breastfeeding was also much longer in both groups of mothers who initiated breastfeeding at or later than one hour after delivery.

TABLE 6-1   Timing of First Effective Breastfeed (IBFAT Score) by Time of Initiation of Breastfeeding and Timing of Labor Medication (N = 43)

	Time of Initiation of Breastfeeding	
Timing of Medications	"Early" < one hour	"Late" > one hour
None / < one hour before birth	Effective BF at 6.4 hours (N = 8)	Effective BF at 49.7 hours (N = 19)
> One hour before birth	Effective BF at 50.3 hours (N = 9)	Effective BF at 62.5 hours (N = 7)

Adapted from: Crowell, et al., 1994.

Local Anesthesia

One study investigated what has been considered a benign intervention as far as the fetus is concerned: local pain medication injected into the vaginal outlet for episiotomy.[23] The timing of 1–2% lidocaine infiltration prior to delivery was investigated in relationship to the ensuing presence of plasma concentrations of this medicine in the newborn after birth. These authors studied 15 normal mothers and their full-term infants. At the time of local infiltration of lidocaine for episiotomy, samples of maternal blood were drawn at seven increments ranging between 1 and 30 minutes. At birth an umbilical vein sample was taken from a singly clamped cord. Finally, maternal and infant blood and urine samples were taken and analyzed at 24 and 48 hours postpartum. Authors found that peak maternal plasma concentrations of lidocaine occur 3-15 minutes after administration, that there is rapid and significant placental transfer, and that lidocaine and its metabolite are found in neonatal urine for up to 48 hours after exposure. Of particular note in their discussion is that the mean fetal/maternal ratio of lidocaine following local perineal infiltration was significantly higher (1.32) than the fetal/maternal ratios previously reported after lumbar epidural for vaginal delivery (0.56) or for cesarean section (0.66).

Lidocaine (commercial names Xylocaine, Lignocaine) is commonly used worldwide for providing local pain relief for the cutting and repair of episiotomy. Although evidence does not support this practice, episiotomy is still routinely cut on all first-time mothers in most of Africa and Asia and is still the most common obstetrical surgical procedure performed in the United States (see Chapter 8). The Phillipson, et al. study discussed above does not link lidocaine use for episiotomy directly with breastfeeding outcomes, but it does establish that the medicine is absorbed by the fetus and remains in the newborn's circulation. Other studies do link lidocaine use in epidurals with impact on breastfeeding. The fact that these authors found that the concentrations of lidocaine are higher with local administration argues for discretionary use of local lidocaine for perineal anesthesia prior to delivery, and reinforces the need to stop all routine use of episiotomy (Figure 6-1).

Epidural Anesthesia

In North America, Europe, and in private facilities that cater to the middle class on all continents, pain medication during labor is

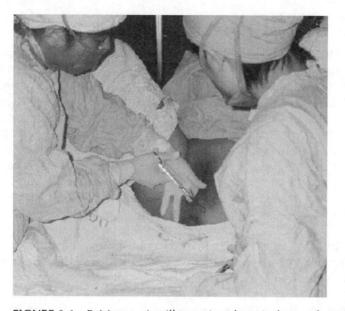

FIGURE 6-1   Episiotomy is still a routine obstetrical procedure worldwide. After injection into the mother's perineum, local anesthesic rapidly enters the maternal bloodstream, crosses the placenta, and reaches the fetus. Traces of this medicine are found in newborn urine at 48 hours of age. *Photo by Mary Kroeger, Beijing, China, 1997.*

increasingly available and clients are prepared to pay for it. The nature of this medicine has changed considerably since the early 1960s, and in the last two decades of the twentieth century in industrialized countries it has become the most commonly available labor anesthesia.[24] Injected into the epidural space of the lumbar vertebrae, this anesthesia has the advantage over earlier spinal anesthetics in that the mother remains completely conscious during labor, while experiencing nearly complete anesthesia from the waist down to her knees or toes. The disadvantages are that the woman usually has to remain in bed, has an intravenous drip, may require a urinary catheter, and in developed country settings, will be constantly attached to electronic fetal monitoring.

Besides its effectiveness in pain relief, one of the biggest selling points of epidural anesthesia to mothers in labor has been that it would have negligible effects on the infant. Evidence is growing that this is not the case. Here again most of the research has been on general neurobehavioral effects on the newborn, but more recently investigators are studying impact on breastfeeding behaviors.

Walker, a nurse/lactation consultant, reviewed thirteen studies, spanning 1981–1995, that had investigated the use of epidural analgesia in labor and infant neurobehavioral outcomes.[25] Selection criteria for studies to be included were: 1) breastfeeding or infant feeding as an outcome, 2) utilization of feeding assessment tools, 3) inclusion of a nonmedicated control group, and 4) assessment of newborn behavior after 24 hours. Unfortunately, none of the studies met all of these criteria. Only five of the studies included nonmedicated controls and only two included assessments of infant behavior after 24 hours of age. No reports included breastfeeding specifically as an outcome. In making comparisons across studies, Walker's discussion articulates the difficulties and the confounding factors in some of the studies, particularly the variation in use of medicines, doses, and timing of administration. Also, the method of delivery, exclusion of babies with fetal distress, and differences in postpartum care all confounded comparisons across studies. In spite of these weaknesses in research design, the author notes that infant behavior was affected by epidural in 7 of the 13 studies, with some infants affected up to one month postpartum. She found that two studies included unmedicated controls and assessed newborn neurobehavior after 24 hours,[26-27] and these are discussed in more detail in the following paragraphs.

Sepkowski and her research team looked prospectively at the effects of epidural anesthesia in labor and its effect on neonatal behavior.[26] Their sample, taken from 60 mothers who vaginally delivered full-term healthy infants, included 22 infants from unmedicated delivery and 38 from epidural delivery. Mothers who had received any other form of labor anesthetic were excluded from the study. Newborn behaviors were assessed by a trained observer who was blind to the medication profile of the mother in labor. The BNBAS was administered four times: at 3 hours after delivery, and on days 3, 7, and 28 postpartum. At the 28-days assessment done in the mother's home, the mother completed a self-esteem questionnaire. Results showed that newborns in the epidural group were less alert and their orientation and motor behavior was significantly more disorganized, with the dose of the medicine used (bupivacaine) related to the mean orientation and motor cluster scores. After controlling for confounding variables, such as long labor, instrumental delivery, and oxytocin augmentation, this effect was statistically significant in the first four days of the newborn's life and continued throughout the first postpartum month. As a secondary finding of this study, the epidural group of mothers was found to have longer labors, more oxytocin augmentations, and more instrumental deliveries than the nonmedicated group. No differences were found in the self-esteem measured at one month, but mothers in the epidural group spent less time with their infants while in hospital, perhaps because they had longer, more difficult deliveries or were recovering from the anesthetic.

Murray and associates in Australia conducted their research on epidurals and newborn behavior a decade earlier than Sepkowski et al.[27] Cohorts in this study were small and included three groups of mothers; one with little or no medication (N = 15), one group that received bupivacaine epidurals (N = 20), and one group with epidurals plus oxytocin augmentation in labor (N = 20). These researchers also used the BNBAS to assess newborn behavior at 24 hours, 5 days, and one month of age. It is not clear if the BNBAS assessors were blind to which study group mother-baby pairs fell in at the time of observations. Findings were that the effects of the epidurals were strongest on day one postpartum and that by day 5 there was behavioral recovery, except that the medicated babies continued to have poor "state organization" as described in the BNBAS. At one month there was little behavioral difference in the babies, but mothers who had not received medication reported their babies to be "more sociable, rewarding and easy to care for," and these mothers were observed to be more responsive to their babies' cries.

A well-designed study on medication in labor and its impact on breastfeeding was done in the United States.[28] These researchers conducted a prospective, blinded, controlled study with a convenience sample of 129 mother-baby pairs who were followed for six weeks postpartum. In such a study it is not possible to randomly assign mothers to certain labor pain medication in labor, and so all mothers meeting selection criteria were included. The IBFAT tool was used to assess infant feeding behavior, thus the parameters used for qualifying breastfeeding effectiveness included readiness to feed, rooting, fixing, and sucking. Each of these four items was graded from 0-3 with a total score of 12 possible. The evaluators were nurses trained as lactation consultants, and they were blinded as to the anesthesia management during labor. Results showed that IBFAT scores were statistically higher in the mothers who had been unmedicated (Figure 6-2). There was no significant difference in duration of breastfeeding between the medicated and unmedicated groups at six weeks postpartum. However, when IBFAT scores were examined across all groups, a low IBFAT score (0–4) was correlated to earlier weaning.

Two publications by Swedish midwives Matthiesen and Ransjo-Arvidson have added to the literature on labor medication and

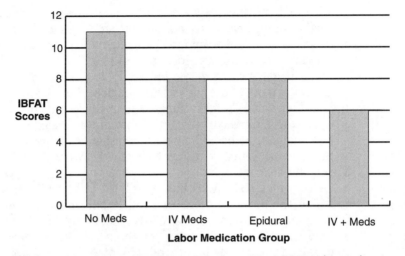

FIGURE 6-2   Onset of Effective Breastfeeding (IBFAT SCORE) by Medication Group Adapted from Figure 1 (Adjusted mean IBFAT score by medicated group) of Riodan J, Gross A, Angeron J, Krumweide B, Melin J. The Effect of Labor Pain Relief Medication on Neonatal Suckling and Breastfeeding Duration. *J Hum Lact* 16(1), 2000.[28]

breastfeeding. The first study observed and described "inborn" feeding behavior in ten unmedicated newborns placed skin to skin with their mothers immediately after delivery.[29] Through careful analysis of videotaped observations, they found that newborns used their hands to explore and stimulate their mother's breasts with a "coordinated pattern of infant hand and sucking movements." When the infants were suckling, the massage-like hand movements stopped and started again when the infants made a sucking pause. These authors found a high significance in the increased maternal oxytocin levels during the periods of increased massage-like hand movements and during actual sucking.

In a second observational study, this research group looked at the impact of various types of labor medication on this apparent inborn feeding behavior.[30] Twenty-eight healthy mothers with uncomplicated pregnancies, vaginal deliveries, and healthy term newborns were included in the study. Immediately after delivery the newborns were dried and put skin to skin on the mothers' chests. Ten mothers had unmedicated labors, six medicated mothers had pudendal block, and 12 mothers had been medicated with both epidural and IV analgesia. The interaction of babies with mothers was videotaped and observers who were blinded to the mothers' labor medication profile recorded specific prefeeding and feeding behaviors. Results showed that all infants made finger and hand movements, but the massage-like movements were less frequent in babies whose mothers' had been medicated. In the epidural group, a significant number of babies made hand-to-mouth movements, and in both the medicated groups there was significantly less touching of the nipple, licking, and actual sucking at the breast (Table 6-2). In other findings, significantly more of the babies from medicated mothers cried longer and had elevated temperatures, compared to the nonmedicated group. These authors conclude that labor anesthesia disturbs a natural behavioral sequence of newborn breast-seeking behavior, adding to the evidence already discussed from the work of Righard and Nissen and colleagues.

A very recent study by Baumgardner et al., 2003[31] has further added to the growing concern about labor epidural and breast-feeding impact. Standarized records were analyzed of two groups of healthy vaginally delivered mothers, 115 of whom received epidural anesthesia in labor and 116 of whom did not. Breast-feeding outcome was measured by 2 successful breastfeedings sessions in the first 24 hours of age as measured by a previously validated method. The mother-baby dyads who received an epidural showed 69.6% successful breastfeeding behavior in the first day postpartum, compared to 81% of mother-baby dyads

TABLE 6-2   Median Time (in Minutes) of First Appearance of Selected Feeding Behaviors in Infants from Medicated and Unmedicated Births

Behavior	No Analgesia (n = 10)	Pudendal Block (n = 6)	Epidural, Pethidine, or Combination of Analgesia (n = 12)
1st opening of eyes	6	5	7
1st breast massage-like movements	11	16	11
1st hand-to-mouth movement	12	21	>120
1st rooting movements	21	20	15
1st hand-to-nipple movement	25	>120	>120
1st licking	27	20	>120
1st sucking	80	>120	>120

Adapted from Ransjö-Arvidson, et al., 2001. Table 4 from Ransjö-Arvidson, et al., Maternal Analgesia During Labor Disturbs Newborn Behavior: Effects on Breastfeeding, Temperature, and Crying. Birth 28:1 March 2001. © 2001 Blackwell Scientific Science, Inc. Used with permission.

who had not received an epidural. Babies of mothers who had an epidural were also more likely to receive a supplementary bottle of formula during their hospital stay.

Labor Medication in Developing Countries and Resource-Poor Settings

The use of labor pain–relieving medicines is not routine in most maternity hospitals in underdeveloped and resource-poor countries. Likewise, in the homebirth setting, mothers do not expect pain medicine, although locally available herbal relaxants in teas or infusions may be offered. In the author's experience in conducting in-service training for practicing midwives in parts of Africa, Central America, Central Asia, and Southeast Asia, midwives in maternity facilities are often unfamiliar with labor pain management techniques other than that provided by medicines. This is in contrast to the author's experience training "traditional" village midwives, who, along with the female relatives of the laboring mother, use pain relief measures such as massage, positioning, warm baths, and prayer. The discussion in Chapter 3 of the positive impact of continuous labor support on many labor outcomes, including lowering perception of pain and lowering actual use of analgesia and anesthesia, argues for the introduction of this intervention in any setting.

The absence of routine labor analgesia and anesthesia in resource-poor settings does not mean that nonpharmacologic interventions cannot be tried. The WHO *Guide for Midwives and Doctors*[20] recommends mobility, position changes, massage, sponging, breathing, and/or a warm bath or shower as possible ways to ease labor pain. Childbirth attendants in any setting should be knowledgeable about these interventions for labor pain relief. As with so many Western obstetrical practices, the use of labor pain medicines in labor will likely increase in resource-poor countries, particularly as poorer countries strive to build capacity for safe deliveries in formal facilities. The rapidly rising cesarean section rates in many countries, discussed more thoroughly in Chapter 8, suggest that increasing numbers of infants will be exposed to medication during births. In countries where extended breastfeeding is still the cultural norm and is essential for both health and economic reasons, the move towards Western labor

pain management methods will be problematic, just as the introduction of infant formula has had a negative impact on infant and
maternal health.

Nonpharmacologic Methods of Pain Relief

Scientific research on nonpharmacologic methods of reducing
labor pain and their impact on labor, delivery, and the newborn
are limited. Continuous support in labor (Chapter 3) is the most
studied and most accepted method. A systematic review of five
methods of labor pain relief and provision of comfort measure
was done by Simkin and O'Hara as one of the contributing papers
presented at the labor pain symposium.[32] Five nonpharmacologic
methods were studied using published randomized controlled
trails (RCT) as the basis for review. These methods were continuous labor support (9 RCTs), baths (7 RCTs and 2 prospective cohort
studies), touch and massage (2 RCTs), maternal movement and
positioning (7 RCTs), and intradermal water blocks for back pain
relief (4 RCTs). Reviews showed that all 5 methods may be effective in reducing labor pain and improving other obstetric out-

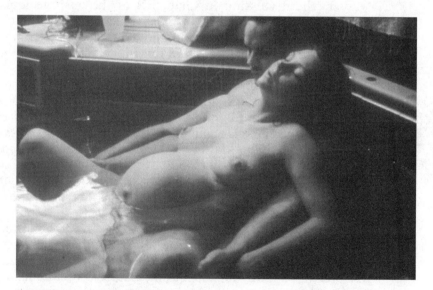

FIGURE 6-3 Hydrotherapy for labor pain relief has been shown to be safe,
to reduce maternal anxiety, to decrease the need for labor anesthesia and
analgesia, and to decease the need for episiotomy. *Photo source CIMS with
permission from Robbie Davis-Floyd.*

comes, and they are safe when used appropriately. Simkin and O'Hara conclude:

> Despite the need for further research, we know enough about these simple and effective methods to recognize that laboring women should have both the opportunity and the encouragement from staff to use them. They are safe, effective, and satisfying for many women, *but are generally unavailable or underutilized because of almost total reliance on a limited variety of pharmacologic methods of pain relief* [author's emphasis added].

Conclusions

This chapter has discussed a few key articles among a very large literature on labor medicines that focus on outcomes in the mother, newborn, breastfeeding behaviors, and breastfeeding. The case has been made that labor pain medicines of all kinds in labor can have adverse effects. The potential side effects of narcotics are clearly established. A finger now must be pointed at epidural anesthesia. The consensus of the 2001 labor pain symposium on in New York is that there are significant adverse labor outcomes associated with epidurals.[33] Two papers presented at the symposium, based on rigorous literature reviews, found evidence that epidural anesthetics can lead to poor childbirth outcomes. These include progress of labor (particularly in first-time mothers), the need for oxytocin augmentation, a longer second stage, a lower rate of spontaneous vaginal delivery, a higher rate of instrumental vaginal delivery, increased maternal fever, and increased evaluation and treatment of newborns for suspected sepsis.[34,35] An earlier review implicated the epidural as being associated with increased cesarean section rates.[36] Using the cascade analogy, it follows that longer, more difficult labors, instrumental and surgical deliveries, and maternal and neonatal fevers in and of themselves bring adverse sequel for mother and newborn. In addition are the possible negative effects of the medications. Yet, in spite of the evidence showing that epidural anesthetics are not benign as a labor intervention, their use in the United States and worldwide is on the increase. The National Maternity Center Survey reports 63% of all mothers surveyed had epidurals in labor.[37] This is a dramatic increase from the 29% of all labor patients in the United States cited in the King review done a few years earlier. The same survey shows 30% of all women surveyed received narcotics in labor as well. The Lieberman and O'Donoghue paper[33] also notes that only two studies they reviewed included breastfeeding as an outcome and these authors did not discuss whether mothers who had received epidural had received narcotics as well. They speculate that opioids and epidural may have "similar effects" on breastfeeding and "there clearly is a need for further research on effects of both epidural and opioid on breast-feeding success."

There is a vast chasm between cumulative research evidence and safe practice when it comes to labor pain medications. Like the suffragists in the 1930s, contemporary childbirth consumers will need to assist clinicians in framing the future direction of labor pain relief. Mothers everywhere have a right to be informed about all possible effects of labor drugs on themselves, their births, their babies, and breastfeeding. Breastfeeding care providers in particular need to recognize that a baby from a medicated birth may begin breastfeeding with clear disadvantages. Education to the mother during pregnancy about breastfeeding must include evidenced-based, honest information about labor drugs. Alternative pain relief measures, with positive birth and breastfeeding outcomes, must be promoted and given the same attention in routine obstetric practice and research agendas.

Summary for Protecting the Mother-Baby Continuum

- Strong evidence exists that meperidine (Demerol, Pethidine) as a labor drug leads to central nervous system depression in the fetus and newborn and negatively impacts breastfeeding. Timing and dose are correlated with effects.
- Strong evidence exists from randomized controlled clinical trails that epidural anesthesia can lead to poor progress of labor (particularly in first-time mothers), need for oxytocin augmentation, a longer second stage, a lower rate of spontaneous vaginal delivery, a higher rate of instrumental vaginal delivery, increased maternal fever, and increased evaluation and treatment of newborns for suspected sepsis.
- Observational evidence shows that epidural and narcotic analgesia affects inborn feeding behaviors and adversely impacts breastfeeding.
- Mothers need to be fully informed of the risks and side effects of labor medicines to the childbirth process, the newborn, and breastfeeding success. Alternative, nonpharmacologic labor pain

relief measures need to be routinely offered as methods of pain relief in labor, and maternity care providers need to be trained in their use.

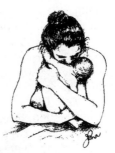

References

1. Wertz D, Wertz R. 1977. *Lying-in: A History of Childbirth in America*. New York: Free Press.
2. Caton D, Frolich MA, Euliana T. 2002. Anesthesia for childbirth: Controversy and change. *Am J Obstet Gynecol*, 186:S25–30.
3. Goland RS, Wardlaw SL, et al. 1981. Human plasma beta-endorphin during pregnancy, labor, and delivery. *J Clin Endocrin Metabolism*, 52(1):74–78.
4. Cahill CA. 1989. Beta-endorphin levels during pregnancy and labor: A role in pain modulation? *Nursing Research*, 38(4):200–203.
5. Robertson A. 1988. *Teaching Active Birth*. Forest Lodge, Australia: Ace Graphics.
6. Brazelton TB. 1961. Effect of maternal medication on the neonate and his behavior. *J Pediatr*, 58(4):513–518.
7. Brazelton TB.1973. Neonatal Behavioral Assessment Scale. In: *Clinics in Developmental Medicine*, No. 50. London: Spastics International Medical Publications.
8. Apgar V. 1966. The newborn (Apgar) scoring system. *Pediatr Clin Am*, 13:645.
9. Scanlon JW, Brown WV, Weiss JB. 1974. Neurobehavioral responses of newborn infants after maternal epidural anesthesia. *Anesthesiology*, 40:121–128.
10. Matthews MK. 1989. The relationship between maternal labour analgesia and delay in the initiation of breastfeeding in healthy neonate in the early neonatal period. *Midwifery*, 5:3–10.

11. Riordan J. 1999. Via Christi breastfeeding assessment tool. Unpublished.

12. Riordan J. 2000. *The Effect of Labor Epidurals on Breastfeeding.* Schaumburg, Illinois: La Leche League International Lactation Consultant Series Two, Unit 4 (No. 298-4).

13. Kuhnert B, Linn Pl, Kenard MJ, et al. 1985. Effects of low doses of meperidine on neonatal behavior. *Int Anesthe Analg,* 64:335–342.

14. Belsey EM, Rosenblatt DB, Lieberman BA, et al. 1981. The influence of maternal analgesia on neonatal behavior: I Pethidine. *Br J Obstet Gynaecol,* 88:398–406.

15. Belfrage P, Boreus LO, Hartvig P, et al. 1981. Neonatal depression after obstetrical analgesia with pethidine. The role of injection-delivery time interval, and the plasma concentrations of pethidine and norpethidine. *Acta Obstet Gynaecol Scand,* 60:43–49.

16. Righard L, Alade MO. 1990. Effect of delivery room routines on success of first breast-feed. *Lancet,* 336:1105–1107.

17. Righard L, Frantz K. 1992. Delivery Self Attachment. Video. Sunland, California: Geddes Productions.

18. Nissan E, Lilja G, Matthiesen AS, et al. 1996. Effects of maternal pethidine on infants' developing breastfeeding behavior. *Research,* 4(2):73–78.

19. Rajan L. 1994. The impact of obstetric procedures and analgesia/anesthesia during labour and delivery on breastfeeding. *Midwifery,* 10:87–103.

20. WHO, UNFPA, UNICEF, World Bank. 2000. *Managing Complications in Pregnancy and Childbirth: A Guide for Midwives and Doctors.* Geneva: World Health Organization. Department of Reproductive Health and Research C-59.

21. Bricker L and Lavender T. 2002. Parenteral opioids for labor-pain relief: A systematic review. *Am J Obstet Gynecol,* 186:S94–109.

22. Crowell MK, Hill PD, Humenick SS.1994. Relationship between obstetric analgesia and time of effective feeding. *Nurse Midwifery* 39(3):150–156.

23. Philipson EH, Kuhnert BR, Syracuse CD. 1984. Maternal, fetal, and neonatal lidocaine levels following local perineal infiltration. *Am J Obstet Gynecol,* 149:403–407.

24. Simchak M. 1991. Has epidural anesthesia made childbirth education obsolete? *Childbirth Instructor,* Summer:15–18.

25. Walker M. 1997. Do labor medications affect breastfeeding? *J of Human Lact,* 13:131–137.

26. Sepkowski C, Lester B, Ostheimer G, Brazelton TB. 1992. The effects of maternal epidural anesthesia on neonatal behavior during the first month. *Devel Med Child Neurol,* 34:1072–1080.

27. Murray AD, Dolby RM, Nation RL, et al. 1981. Effects of epidural anesthesia on newborns and their mothers. *Child Development,* 53:71–82.

28. Riordan J, Gross A, Angeron J, et al. 2000. The effect of labor pain relief medication on neonatal suckling and breastfeeding duration. *J of Human Lact*, 16 (1):7–12.

29. Matthiesen A, Ransjo-Arvidson A, Gunilla L, et al. 2001. Postpartum maternal oxytocin release by newborns: Effects of infant hand massage and suckling. *Birth*, 28(1):13–19.

30. Ransjo-Arvidson A, Matthiesen A, Gunilla L, et al. 2001. Maternal analgesia during labor disturbs newborn behavior: Effects on breastfeeding, temperature, and crying. *Birth*, 28(1):5–12.

31. Baumgarder DJ, Muehl P, Fisher M, et al. 2003. Effect of epidural anesthesia on breastfeeding of healthy fullterm newborns delivered vaginally. *J Am Board Fam Pract*, 16(1):7–13.

32. Simkin P, O'Hara M, 2002. Nonpharmacolgic relief of pain during labor: Systematic reviews of five methods. *Am J Obstet Gynecol*, 186:S131–159.

33. Rooks JP, Sakala C, Corry MP, Eds. 2002. *The Nature and Management of Labor Pain:* Peer-reviewed Papers from an Evidence-based Symposium. New York: Mosby, Inc. 2002.

34. Lieberman E and O'Donoghue C, 2002. Unintended effects of epidural analgesia during labor: A systematic review. *Am J Obstet Gynecol*, 186: S31–68.

35. Leighton BL, Halpern SH. 2002. The effects of epidural analgesia on labor, maternal and neonatal outcomes: A systematic review. *Am J Obstet Gynecol*, 186:S69–77.

36. King T. 1997. Epidural anesthesia in labor: Benefits versus risks. *J Nurse Midwifery*, 42(5):377–391.

37. Declercq ER, Sakala C, Corry MP, Applebaum S, Risher P. 2002. *Listening to Mothers: Report of the First National U.S. Survey of Women's Childbearing Experiences*, New York: Maternity Center Association October 2002, *www.maternity.org/listeningto mothers/results.html*.

CHAPTER 7

PHYSICS, FORCES, AND MECHANICAL EFFECTS OF BIRTH ON BREASTFEEDING

by Linda J. Smith

"Whenever a body exerts a force on another body, the latter exerts a force of equal magnitude and opposite direction on the former."

Sir Isaac Newton, 1687

Obstetric textbooks sometimes describe childbirth as a process involving the three "P's": the power, the passenger, and the passage. This chapter discusses these three concepts in the context of breastfeeding outcomes. As postpartum care providers, including lactation consultants, become more experienced and skilled in helping mothers to breastfeed, a pattern of problems is becoming evident among healthy term infants. These problems are clearly infant-related issues seen in otherwise healthy babies, and include the following:

- Babies who can latch but cannot sustain sucking
- Babies who appear to suck, but cannot transfer or obtain milk from a full breast
- Babies who cannot smoothly coordinate sucking, swallowing, and breathing
- Babies who can feed in only one position or posture
- Babies who are dissatisfied at breast and fussy or distressed many hours per day
- Babies who chew, crease, and damage the mothers' nipple(s)
- Babies who may not feed much better from devices

These situations are not related to maternal motivation, family or social stresses, or unrealistic expectations of infant behavior. Nor are these primarily breast problems. However, if the situation is not resolved, milk stasis in the mother's breast quickly compromises milk synthesis[1] and/or causes nipple damage.[2] Possible contributing factors include epidural anesthesia/analgesia, forceps delivery, vacuum extraction, induction of labor, Cesarean delivery, or long, difficult labor, especially with occiput posterior positioning. The baby may have visible cranial or postural asymmetry secondary to these interventions or may appear to be normal.

The rates of many childbirth interventions are rapidly exceeding the legitimate indications for their use in many areas, both in the United States and worldwide. There is no "smoking gun" research that clearly explains why some otherwise healthy, full-term babies cannot suck normally after operative or medicated births. The few studies that even mention breastfeeding at all consider "still breastfeeding at 6 weeks" as evidence to support the allegation that interventions and medications are innocuous.[3] The fact that so many mothers and babies can manage to establish and maintain breastfeeding despite early problems related to medications or mechanically assisted births is a testament to excellent postbirth support. However, the challenges mothers and babies face in those six weeks can be very daunting (see Box 7-1).

Box 7-1 Case History of a Baby with Persistent Poor Suck

Annie called the lactation consultant (LC) when Jared was 7 weeks old because Jared was barely gaining weight, her nipples were still cracked and bleeding, and breastfeeding was "very difficult and deteriorating." She wanted to breastfeed Jared at least a full year because of diabetes in her family. At 37.5 weeks gestation, her labor was induced with Pitocin and an epidural containing bupivicaine and fentanyl was started. 17 hours later she was fully dilated and began to push; 2 1/2 hours later, Jared was delivered with vacuum extractor. His APGAR scores were 6 and 8 at 1 and 5 minutes respectively. He was suctioned with a bulb syringe, placed in a radiant warmer for 2 hours, and then reunited with Annie in the recovery room where she tried to breastfeed for the first time. Jared appeared "groggy and disoriented" and did not latch, but she kept trying for the next few hours. Exhausted, she allowed the nurses to take Jared to the nursery where he was given 2 oz. glucose water but immediately gagged and vomited the feed. She kept him nearby and continued to attempt latching; several nurses helped her position him better, with not much success. By 24 hours he was still not latching. Becoming concerned, Annie started expressing colostrum to feed Jared in a spoon. The next day he was taking 10 cc of colostrum by spoon every 2 hours, but still not latching, and he continued to gag.

Annie went home, even more worried because Jared was beginning to look yellow and had not stooled since birth. On day 3, Annie's milk supply was rapidly increasing and Jared was taking about 30 cc every hour by spoon, and had begun to latch on the right breast a few times. He had three wet diapers and a small black stool that day. At breast, he gagged and choked during her let-down, stopped and started, and after 40 minutes seemed to get some milk; afterward, Annie's nipples were creased and painful. Annie rented an electric breast pump, and was tempted to use formula so she could get some rest. By day 4, Jared was still struggling at breast, but was more alert and stooling more. Annie's nipples felt very painful, and Jared could still feed only on the right side. Feeds were long and difficult for both of them. At a pediatric checkup on day 5, Jared's doctor pronounced him healthy even though Annie was very concerned that he was not feeding well and his head was flat on one side.

Their mutual struggle continued. Annie pumped every 2-3 hours to get milk and cup fed Jared the pumped milk. She suffered through mind-numbing fatigue. Her continued attempts at direct breastfeeding deteriorated into frustrating 45-minute struggles, ending when until Annie's nipple pain became unbearable. Jared's slow weight gain and very unhappy cries for another 6 weeks convinced Annie to seek more help. The LC corrected the way Annie held Jared, which helped a little on the right breast, but Jared still couldn't manage nursing comfortably on the left and did not tolerate any touch deep in his mouth, where her nipple should have rested during feeds. The LC continued working with Annie and Jared another three weeks until Annie felt Jared was nursing "good enough." He still had a flattened area on his head, gagged and choked during feeds, and only fed comfortably in one position. At 5 months of age, Annie contacted the LC to say she had given up even trying to nurse directly, and continued to pump for another several months. By 8 months, Jared was completely weaned to formula and bottles. Annie called the LC one last time, saying she was sad, frustrated, and depressed because Jared suffered from pneumonia twice since he weaned, still gags on most solid food, and has not yet begun crawling.

Breastfeeding cessation rates are highest in the first few weeks after birth. Rates of hospital readmission for breastfed babies for hyper-bilirubinemia, dehydration, and other feeding-related illnesses have increased in the United States.[4,5] Many professionals are questioning whether undocumented and poorly researched infant-related feeding difficulties are partly responsible for these problems.[6] This chapter takes what is known about infant cranial anatomy, the physiology of suck-swallow-breathe coordination, and the birth process, and explores a connection with research findings.

Nerves and Muscles Control Movement

Humans are the most immature mammal offspring at birth, requiring the longest postbirth developmental period, which anthropologist Ashley Montague describes as the period of "exterogestation."[7] The human infant's skull (cranium) is the tightest "fit" of all mammals as it passes through the mother's pelvis (see Figure 7-1). During birth, the infant's head and body must pass through the bony pelvis or be pulled out through an incision in the mother's uterus and abdomen. Normal birth, for the

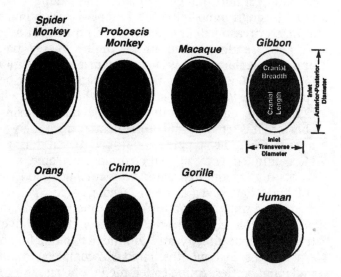

FIGURE 7-1 Diagram of the size of the neonate's head (black oval) relative to the pelvic outlet. Rosenberg, K., Trevathan, W., "Bipedalism and human birth: the obstetrical dilemma revisited." *Evolutionary Anthropology* 4(5): 161–168. 1996. Reprinted by permission of Wiley-Liss, Inc., a subsidiary of John Wiley & Sons, Inc.

purposes of this chapter, is defined as spontaneous birth of a full-term infant over the mother's intact perineum.

Birth affects the infant mechanically, physically, physiologically, pharmacologically, neurologically, and nutritionally. For breastfeeding to succeed, the baby must be able and willing to feed, the mother must be able and willing to let her baby nurse, the process should be comfortable and pleasant for both, and circumstances and surroundings must support the dyad so the mother feels free to continue. Infant feeding ability requires:

- A patent, uncompromised airway
- Oropharyngeal muscle patterns, coordination, and strength sufficient to obtain milk from the lactating breast
- Psychomotor ability to signal the need to feed.[9]

A baby who is compromised in any of these dynamic systems is at risk for feeding problems.

Breastfeeding Is Movement

Physical movement is accomplished by muscles controlled by nerves acting on bones. Sucking, swallowing, and breathing are no exception. The infant skull consists of 22 bones that articulate at 34 sutures/joints. Some of these bony segments fuse early in infancy (for example, the two pieces of the frontal bone); others remain open (connected by fibrous sutures) into adulthood. Motor nerves control some 60 voluntary and involuntary muscles that move the tongue, jaw, pharynx, epiglottis, respiratory structures, and face.[10] The baby's airway must remain open when appropriate and aligned (patent) throughout the feed.

Feeding involves complex interrelated movement patterns that are controlled and coordinated by 6 of the 12 cranial nerves (V, VII, IX, X, XI, and XII) and 3 cervical cord segments (C1-3) (see Figure 7-2). These have been studied extensively in the context of feeding and swallowing disorders.[11] Sensory fibers in these nerves receive input from the tongue, palate, lips, jaw, and other structures. Breathing overrules sucking—if the baby cannot breathe, the baby will not begin feeding, will stop quickly, or will feed in a disorganized pattern[11] (see Figure 7-3). The first manifestation of an airway problem can be a feeding problem.[12]

The normal infant sucks 40–60 times per minute at a ratio of 1:1:1 (one suck, one swallow, one breath), in bursts of 10–30 sucks followed by a brief pause and resumption of this pattern.[13,11] A normal feed usually falls in the range of 10–30 minutes per breast, and concludes with the infant self-detaching from the breast in

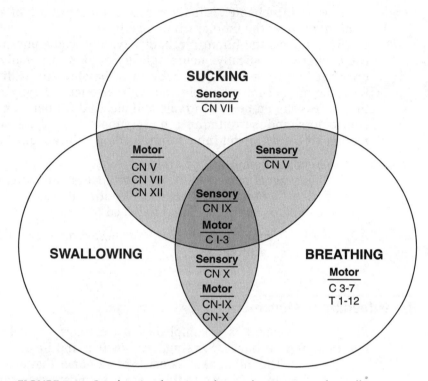

FIGURE 7-2 Overlapping function of cranial nerves in suck-swallow-breathe.[11]

obvious satiation, often at the peak of a let-down reflex.[14] The baby's spontaneous detachment from the breast is a strong indicator of infant self-regulation of milk intake. The baby typically takes about 76% of the milk stored in the breast, even though more is available for the taking.[15]

Cranial Bones Surround the Developing Infant Brain

Normal birth requires molding of the fetal skull with associated shifting of the four segments of the occiput, both parietal bones, and three segments of each temporal bone (see Figure 7-4).[10] The parietal bones override the basilar portion of the occiput and the two halves of the frontal bone, allowing the fetal head to "corkscrew" through the maternal pelvis. After birth, sucking and crying help expand the cranial vault, allowing the bones to gradually move back into alignment over the first 1–2 weeks post-

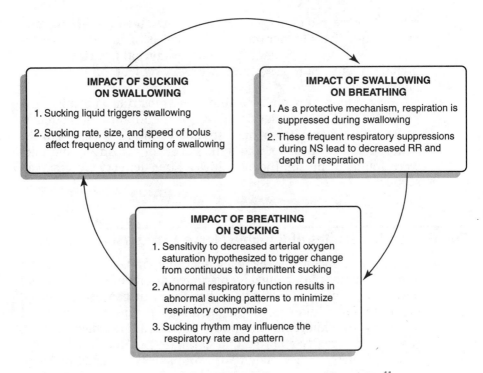

**IMPACT OF SUCKING
ON SWALLOWING**

1. Sucking liquid triggers swallowing

2. Sucking rate, size, and speed of bolus
   affect frequency and timing of swallowing

**IMPACT OF SWALLOWING
ON BREATHING**

1. As a protective mechanism, respiration is
   suppressed during swallowing

2. These frequent respiratory suppressions
   during NS lead to decreased RR and
   depth of respiration

**IMPACT OF BREATHING
ON SUCKING**

1. Sensitivity to decreased arterial oxygen
   saturation hypothesized to trigger change
   from continuous to intermittent sucking

2. Abnormal respiratory function results in
   abnormal sucking patterns to minimize
   respiratory compromise

3. Sucking rhythm may influence the
   respiratory rate and pattern

FIGURE 7-3   Interrelationship of sucking, swallowing, and breathing.[11]

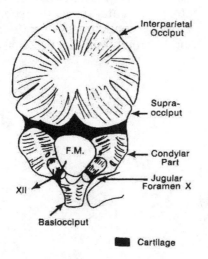

Interparietal
Occiput

Supra-
occiput

Condylar
Part

Jugular
Foramen X

F.M.

XII

Basiocciput

■ Cartilage

FIGURE 7-4   Cranial base showing jugular foramen and hypoglossal
canal.[23]

birth.[16] As the end of pregnancy approaches, the newborn has elevated (three times higher than normal) levels of endogenous beta-endorphins[17,18] which may ameliorate any pain during birth,[19] including any pain associated with movement of the cranial plates.

Beta-endorphins are also found in colostrum and milk, and provide significant analgesic effects to the infant.[20] Researchers in Italy found that labor pain stimulates higher levels of beta-endorphins in colostrum and milk. Levels in colostrum and milk were found to be significantly lower after delivery by cesarean section.[21]

The Cranial Base: Sites of Possible Nerve Entrapment

Cranial asymmetry of the occipital, temporal, and/or parietal bones is often accompanied by disrupted alignment of the cranial base.[22] Cranial asymmetry is a possible cause or contributing factor to short and long term neurological and developmental problems in children.[23] A group of Harvard Medical School researchers recently reported that in the first 1–3 days of life, cranial asymmetry is associated with primiparity, assisted delivery, and long labor (see Figure 7-5a and b). Early posterior cranial flattening or otherwise unusual head shapes can progress to deformational plagiocephaly (asymmetry without suture fusing). Cranial asymmetry is more common in males, twins, and on the right side, and may contribute to postnatal torticollis (shortening of the sternocleidomastoid muscle). Cephalohematoma is a well-known risk factor for posterior deformational plagiocephaly. Mul-

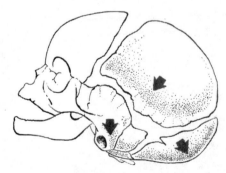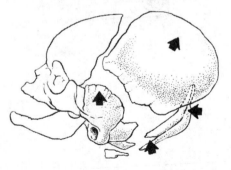

FIGURE 7-5   Diagrams of molding.

tiple births and uterine constraints have been reported as risk factors for plagiocephaly but not true synostosis (fusing of the sutures).[24] Lactation care providers have anecdotally reported that babies with poor suck often have cranial asymmetry.

The hypoglossal nerve (C XII) controls tongue movement, including the patterns necessary for latch and sucking (see Figure 7-6). In the infant, C XII lies in the space between segments of the occipital bone, which later fuse to form the hypoglossal canal in adults. Disruption of the occipital segments could lead to nerve entrapment of the hypoglossal nerve(s), which in turn could cause or contribute to ineffective, mispatterned, and/or disorganized contraction patterns in the tongue muscle group.

Three cranial nerves and the jugular vein pass through the jugular foramen, which lies between the occiputal segments and

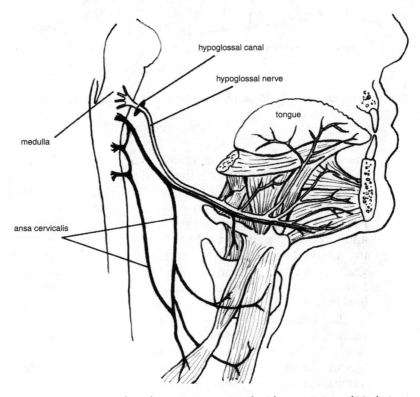

FIGURE 7-6   Hypoglossal nerve (C XII). Used with permission of Linda J. Smith.

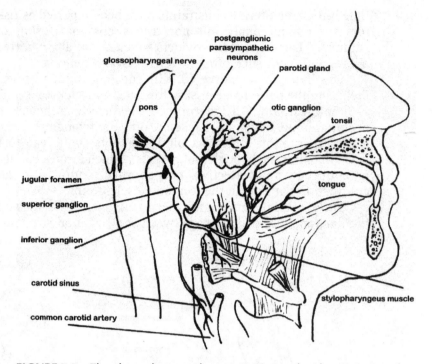

FIGURE 7-7   The glossopharyngeal nerve (C IX). Used with permission of Linda J. Smith.

the temporal bones. The glossopharyngeal nerve (C IX) has sensory fibers in the posterior palate and tongue, which, among other functions, trigger the gag response (see Figure 7-7). Motor fibers control pharyngeal muscles involved in swallowing. A hyper-responsive gag can prevent the infant's deep attachment at breast and force the nipple up against the rugae of the hard palate, causing nipple damage and poor milk transfer.[25] If the glossopharyngeal nerve is compromised, any or all of these sensory or motor functions may be affected, and may adversely affect suck-swallow-breathe and comfortable, coordinated breastfeeding.

The heart, lungs, trachea, bronchi, larynx, pharynx, gastrointestinal tract, and external ear are innervated by sensory fibers of the vagus nerve (C X) (see Figure 7-8). Motor fibers control the larynx, heart, lungs, trachea, liver, and gastrointestinal tract. Some lactation care providers have observed that babies with poor suck may produce a high-pitched squeal during feeds, suggesting laryngeal dysfunction. Coordination of suck with breathing, another function of vagal control, is necessary for effective, com-

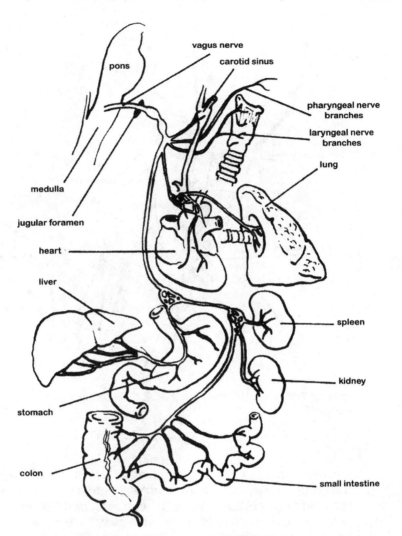

pons

vagus nerve

carotid sinus

pharyngeal nerve
branches

laryngeal nerve
branches

lung

medulla

jugular foramen

heart

liver

spleen

kidney

stomach

colon

small intestine

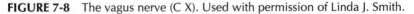

FIGURE 7-8   The vagus nerve (C X). Used with permission of Linda J. Smith.

fortable feeds. Gastroesophageal reflux, also related to vagal function, affects a baby's ability and willingness to breastfeed. If the vagus nerve is compromised, any or all of vagal functions may be affected and adversely affect suck-swallow-breathe and comfortable, coordinated breastfeeding.

Torticollis alone (shortening or spasm of the SCM muscle) or torticollis associated with nerve entrapment from cranial asymmetry,[24] could explain why some babies can feed well in only one position or posture. The trapezius and sternocleidomastoid (SCM)

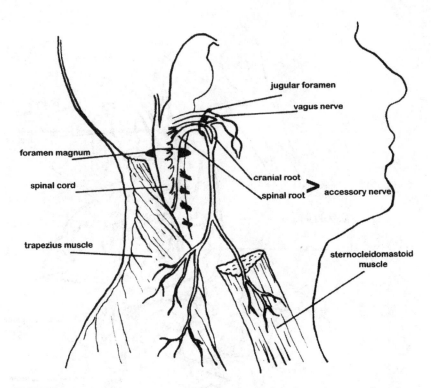

FIGURE 7-9   Spinal Accessory nerve (C XI). Used with permission of Linda J. Smith.

muscles, innervated by the spinal accessory nerve (C XI), stabilize the infant's head and maintain airway patency (see Figure 7-9). If the spinal accessory nerve is compromised, reduced airway patency and torticollis may adversely affect suck-swallow-breathe and comfortable coordinated breastfeeding.

Caput succedaneum is a localized edematous swelling of the scalp caused by the pressure of the dilating cervix against the infant cranium (see Figure 7-10). The jugular vein also passes through the jugular foramen, therefore it follows that disruption or misalignment of the foramen may affect venous return. Caput is a "given" following vacuum extraction. When caput occurs, venous return via the jugular vein and other vessels is obstructed, resulting in edema. One text claims "caput disappears in several days and is of *no pathologic significance.*"[26] (italics added by the author). Lactation care providers have anecdotally reported that babies with caput feed poorly in horizontal positions, and behave

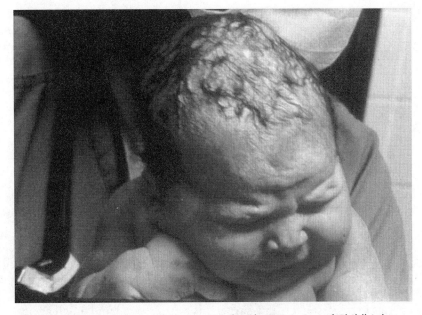

FIGURE 7-10   An infant with caput. Used with permission of Childbirth Graphics.

as if they have a severe headache. If the jugular foramen is disrupted or misaligned by mechanical forces during instrument-assisted birth, then altered function of the jugular vein and the three cranial nerves passing through the foramen may adversely affect suck-swallow-breathe and comfortable, coordinated breastfeeding.

Mechanical Forces and Instruments During Birth

"Deleterious effects of uterine forces upon the fetus during labor and delivery were documented by Little in 1862."[16] Excessive pressures to the fetal head, which can be caused by uterine tetany, forceps delivery, or excessive fundal pressure, can increase fetal intracranial pressure.[27]

Use of a vacuum extractor substantially increases the amount of force applied to the occipital segments and has a documented risk of complications. Hall et al. (2002) studied a large sample of suburban middle-class mothers who intended to breastfeed. Mothers were interviewed prior to birth, and postpartum after hospital discharge. They reported that "Data strongly suggests that success of breastfeeding is associated with events in the first two weeks of life, if not the first 3 to 5 days." Vacuum vaginal delivery was a strong predictor of early cessation of breastfeeding.[28]

Box 7-2   U.S. FDA Public Health Advisory: Need for CAUTION When Using Vacuum Assisted Delivery Devices—May 21, 1998 *www.fda.gov/cdrh/safety.html*[29]

"Although all infants exposed to vacuum assisted delivery devices will have a caput succedaneum, care providers need to be aware that two major life-threatening complications following use of vacuum assisted devices have been reported to us:

Subgaleal hematoma (Subaponeurotic hematoma): This occurs when emissary veins are damaged and blood accumulates in the potential space between the galea aponeurotica (epicranial aponeurosis) and the periosteum of the skull (pericraniaum). Since the subaponeurotic space has no containing membranes nor boundaries, the subgaleal hematoma may extend from the orbital ridges to the nape of the neck. This condition is dangerous because of the large potential space for blood accumulation and the possibility of life-threatening hemorrhage.

Intracranial Hemorrhage: This may include subdural, subarachnoid, intraventricular, and/or intraparenchymal hemorrhage."

Instrument delivery with forceps causes lateral compression of the parietal and three segments of each temporal bone. "Forceps use can cause bruising and nerve damage to the sides of the infant cranium, causing the jaw to deviate to the paralyzed side when the mouth is open"[30] (see Figures 7-11 and 7-12).

Nerves Are Affected by Mechanical Forces

Forceps use can cause damage to the trigeminal nerve (C V), which has sensory fibers to the palate, tongue, lower jaw, and nose (see

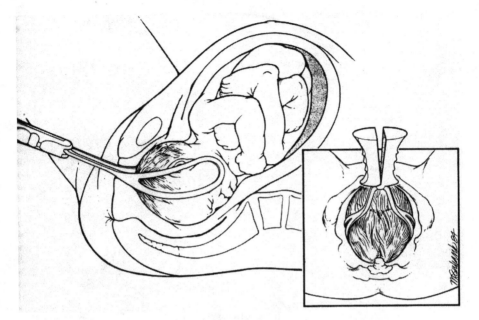

FIGURE 7-11 Application of forceps. Reprinted from Obstetrics: Normal and Problem Pregnancies, 2nd ed. Gabbe SG, Niebyl JR, Simpson JL, eds. Figure 14.7. © 1991. With permission from Elsevier.

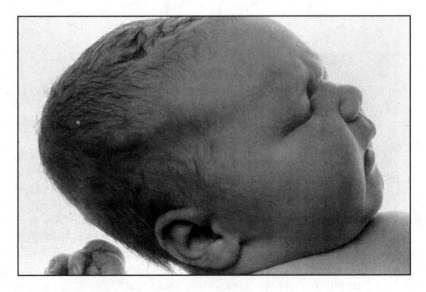

FIGURE 7-12 Baby with forceps bruises. *Source: Childbirth Graphics.*

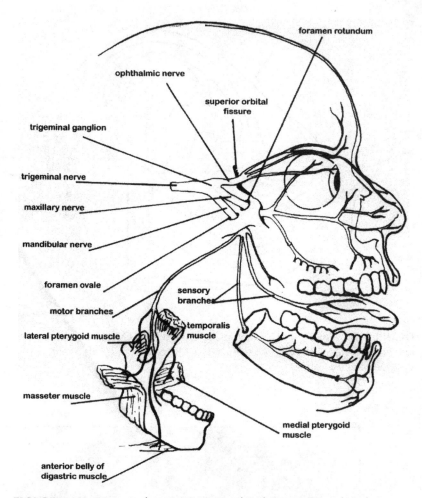

FIGURE 7-13 Trigeminal nerve (C V). Used with permission of Linda J. Smith.

Figure 7-13). Cool air on the infant's face is a trigger for respiration, a sensory response central to suck-swallow-breathe. Motor fibers innervate the muscles that control mouth opening, closing, and sucking (masseter, ptergoid, mentalis, and temporalis). The baby must be able to open the jaw to a wide (>160°) angle to allow deep latch.[31] Vertical (downward) movement of the mandible increases the negative intraoral pressures (suck) drawing the nipple/areolar complex into a long teat.[32] Negative pressures also help propel the milk into the infant's posterior oral space, triggering swallowing. Closing the mandible occurs during swallowing. If the trigeminal nerve is compromised, sensory triggers for respiration and motor control of the mandible may adversely affect suck-swallow-breathe and comfortable, coordinated breastfeeding.

The facial nerve (C VII) has sensory fibers to the palate and anterior two-thirds of the tongue, and is involved in many of the proprioceptive functions of the infant mouth (see Figure 7-14). The infant's suck response is triggered by tactile receptors in the lips and palate. Therefore, the facial nerve must be intact and functioning normally for the baby to begin feeding. Motor fibers control the facial muscles, lips, cheeks, and jaw, which are also directly involved in rooting, latching, and sucking responses. If the facial nerve is compromised, the infant may not be able to feel or respond to the breast in its mouth, nor use the tongue to grasp the nipple-areolar complex. Compromise to the motor fibers could result in using lip muscles to tightly grasp the nipple tip, instead of using tongue and intraoral muscles to grasp the nipple/areolar complex, thereby adversely affecting normal suck-swallow-breathe and comfortable, coordinated breastfeeding.

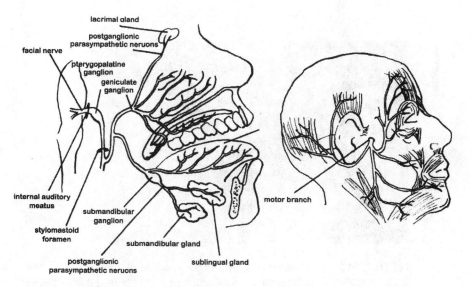

FIGURE 7-14 The facial nerve (C VII). Used with permission of Linda J. Smith.

Physics and Forces During Cesarean Delivery

Lactation care providers have observed more breastfeeding problems in babies born by cesarean birth than in babies born vaginally (see Chapter 8). When a cesarean delivery is performed, the practitioner's fingertips are usually placed under the condylar portions of the occiput bone, and the infant is lifted out of the incision with upward traction on the cranial base (see Figure 7-15).

Consider these facts: The newborn's occiput is in four pieces. The hypoglossal nerve runs between the condylar and basilar portions of the occipital plates, and the jugular foramen is directly adjacent to the condylar portion of the occiput. Therefore, the potential exists for disruption of the jugular foramen, hypoglossal canal, and the nerves and vessels passing through these spaces.

Babies born by cesarean usually require considerable suctioning, because the oralpharyngeal mucus is not squeezed out as it is during vaginal birth. Suctioning and intubation have additional mechanical effects on infant oral motor function. Pediatrician Linda Black observed petechiae and abrasions on the posterior palates of babies who were suctioned after vaginal births using standard bulb syringes.[33] "Lacerations and bruises of pharyngeal and laryngeal structures may result from rough insertion of the laryngoscope. Injury to the larynx is particularly seri-

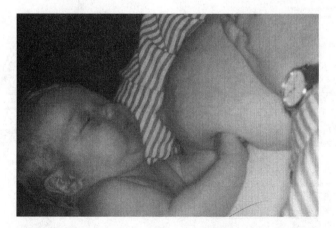

FIGURE 7-15 This baby was delivered by cesarean plus forceps. Note the arching posture and the mother's flattened nipple. At breast, he only chewed and flattened the nipple and could not obtain milk despite the mother's skill and good milk supply. Used with permission of Linda J. Smith.

ous because the airway may be occluded by edema or hemorrhage."[26]

Muscle Responses and Mispatterning

The tongue is a set of muscles (see Figure 7-16). A superstimulus to any muscle group creates neural patterning that is permanent, also known as "muscle memory." To establish other movements in the same muscle group, secondary neuromotor pathways must be established and reinforced. The tongue muscle group can be mispatterned by early superstimuli such as deep or repeated suctioning, which results in posterior-to-anterior peristalsis. Tongue thrusting is a documented consequence of bottle-feeding and pacifier use, and bottle-feeding and pacifier use are known detriments to breastfeeding.[34]

Physical irritation of the posterior palate (innervated by the glossopharyngeal nerve) creates a reflex guarding of the airway by the tongue, which moves forward and up, pressing against the palate. This is exactly the opposite of the anterior-to-posterior tongue peristalsis needed for breastfeeding.[2] This tongue motion prevents the nipple from being drawn deeply into the

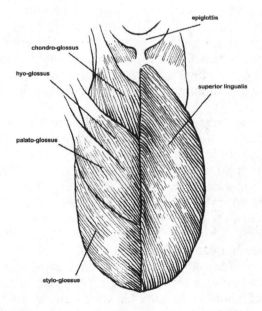

FIGURE 7-16 Tongue muscle groups. Used with permission of Linda J. Smith.

baby's mouth, thereby preventing effective latch, sucking, and milk transfer.

Cesarean births have become epidemic in some places (see Chapter 8), and some physicians even argue for elective primary cesarean sections. Even if the baby were unaffected by the anesthetics and analgesics used and the mother were likewise unaffected by major surgery, the physics and forces affecting the infant adversely affect normal suck-swallow-breathe and comfortable, coordinated breastfeeding.

Effects of Analgesia and Anesthesia on Nerve Function

Chapter 6 covered much of the clinical research on the impact of labor medications on breastfeeding. Most drugs administered to the mother for labor pain relief are highly lipid soluble and designed to affect the mother's sensory nerves. They reach the mother's brain and central nervous system (CNS) quickly and are sequestered in nerve tissue, which is precisely the reason they are effective in reducing or blocking pain.

Concerns about the effects of these drugs on the newborn are not new. Over a century ago, physicians worried about anesthesic's effects on the newborn, and argued that ether not be used for normal deliveries until it could be properly tested. As the use of regional anesthesia increased, "physicians sought the local anesthetics [for use in epidurals] with least affect on the child. Clinicians also sought local anesthetics that inherently had less effect on motor nerves."[35] In a randomized double-blind study, Loftus reaffirmed earlier research establishing rapid placental transfer of drugs (sufentanil, fentanyl, and bupivicane) to the neonate.[36]

Putting these facts together, it is accepted that anesthetics cross the placenta, reach the infant quickly (15 seconds to 2 minutes), are highly lipid soluble, and target the mother's sensory nerve tissue. Therefore, it is entirely possible that these drugs also affect the infant's sensory nerves. If the facial or trigeminal nerves, which innervate the palate and lips, are numbed from anesthetic agents, the infant might not be able to sense the presence of a breast—which could explain the infant who doesn't latch, or latches but cannot sustain sucking.

Randomized controlled studies have established that maternal anesthetic agents also affect motor nerves, resulting in a longer second stage of labor (see Chapter 6). Anesthetic agents also affect the infant's breathing, sucking, and muscle tone. If the facial, trigeminal, spinal accessory, and/or hypoglossal nerves are affected by maternal anesthetic agents, the infant might be unable to effectively coordinate sucking, swallowing, and breathing—which could explain the baby that appears to suck, but cannot transfer or obtain milk from a full breast.

Baumgarder's recent study confirms the type of problems listed at the beginning of this chapter: healthy, full term newborns that attempt to breastfeed but cannot feed normally. Although the authors did not report the number of babies exposed to forceps, vacuum extraction, or induction, they conclude "labor epidural anesthesia had a negative impact on breastfeeding in the first 24 hours of life, even though it did not inhibit the percentage of breast-feeding attempts in the first hour." Whether the inability to latch is because of the medications, mechanical forces, or a combination of factors, is still unknown, the problem is very real.[37]

Implications of Interventions to the Physics of Suck-Swallow-Breathe

Epidural analgesia and/or anesthesia increases the risks of maternal and infant fever, longer first stage of labor, instrument-assisted delivery, cesarean section, infant seizures, and septic workups.[38] Longer labor and instrument use increase the mechanical forces on the infant cranium and nerves. Induction of labor with oxytocin results in stronger uterine contractions, which put more pressure on the baby's presenting part (usually the occiput), increasing the risk of cranial molding, asymmetry, and cranial base misalignment. Induction of labor is sometimes done for less than compelling medical reasons, resulting in a near-term or "borderline" baby[39] with immature or disorganized feeding abilities and a higher risk of readmission to the hospital.

Pharmacological pain relief increases the risk of the infant requiring resuscitation. Infant resuscitation increases the risk of damage to the oropharyngeal tissues and mispatterning of the tongue and muscles involved in suck-swallow-breathe. In addition, infants needing resuscitation are often separated from their mothers.

Newborn complications increase the risk of separation of mother and baby, which is a well-known barrier to establishing breastfeeding.[40] In addition to alterations in oral motor functioning when separation occurs, separated babies cry more.[41] Crying increases risks of postbirth intercranial bleeds.[42] Symptoms of intracranial bleeds in term newborns include hypotonia or hypertonia, disturbed swallowing, disturbed sucking, transient apnea, and tremor or jerks.[43]

Implications of Poor Suck-Swallow-Breathe

If a baby cannot feed effectively, lack of hydration and reduced caloric intake further compromises the sucking response, and a dangerous downward spiral begins. The compromised baby can't feed well, therefore muscle function is weakened and less effective, and the infant becomes more disorganized and even less able to feed. Hypoglycemia and hyperbilirubinemia become a threat. The baby who can't get colostrum is deprived of immune protection, calories, and beta-endorphins found in colostrum and milk, further increasing its pain and physiological and psychological stress.

Babies who cannot breastfeed normally are deprived of a potent and safe analgesic: breastfeeding and breast milk itself.[44,20,21] In addition, sucking is calming to the central nervous system and helps the baby to self-regulate.

Many professionals legitimately ask "how long is too long to wait" to begin supplementing, and the answer is far from clear. Other common unanswered questions include:

- What device should be used to feed the "breastfed" baby who is unable to breastfeed?
- Will use of these devices undermine the mother's confidence, cause "nipple confusion" or mispatterning, and alter milk composition?
- When will the baby recover from these early problems and begin to feed normally?

If the baby cannot feed effectively, another downward cascade related to milk production and postpartum physiological changes begins. Colostrum and milk remain in the breast, causing or exacerbating engorgement and triggering early mammary involution as early as a few days postbirth.[1,45] More unanswered questions include the following:

- If the baby can't feed, when should the mother begin to express or pump milk?
- If the baby is damaging the nipple because of poor suck, how long will the mother persist before quitting in pain?
- What does nipple or breast pain do to the mother's relationship with her baby?
- What techniques or pumps are the most comfortable, effective, and affordable for removing milk?
- What effect will all of these problems have on establishing a mutually satisfying mother-baby relationship?

It is no surprise that babies who cannot feed well at breast are often supplemented. However, supplements do not fix underlying problems affecting suck-swallow-breathe. Left unrecognized and uncorrected, underlying cause(s) of early feeding problems may have long-term consequences. Conversely, early feeding problems may be markers for other pathology in the infant. Furthermore, feeding mother's milk with a device isn't breastfeeding. Milk fed to the infant by a device is different nutritionally and immunologically from that which the infant obtains directly from the mother's breast.[14] Breastfeeding itself is fundamentally different from sucking on other objects and has long-term implications.[46,47] If a normal full-term baby cannot feed at a normal breast, the most urgent and appropriate question to ask is, "What is wrong with the baby?"

For the mother, giving birth to a baby who cannot suck, swallow, and/or breathe normally is usually an enormous shock. Other people (family or healthcare providers) may make matters worse by blaming her, her breasts, or her milk for the baby's problems. She will need additional help, techniques, and/or equipment to collect her milk and feed it to her baby indirectly, further undermining her confidence and possibly compromising her milk supply. Mothers whose babies cannot feed at breast often grieve for months or years afterward.[48] The fundamental mother-baby continuum has been disrupted.

Conclusions

Randomized controlled trials have not looked at these connections. Because of the dearth of research connecting birth practices and breastfeeding, the case being made in this chapter may be difficult to prove. Professionals have just begun to explore these connections. For example, Dr. Maxwell Fraval collaborated with Dr. Peter Hartmann, a renowned lactation researcher in Australia, to measure the results of osteopathic treatment of infants with sucking dysfunction, with encouraging results.[49] Dr. Judith O'Connell et al. submitted a research proposal to the U.S. National Institutes of Health in 1993,[50] but lack of a validated tool to measure changes in infant suck stymied further formal study.

We have taken what is known about anatomy, physiology, endocrinology, and other fields, plus what is known about breastfeeding problems, and suggested "connecting the dots" in a way that has never been done before. More research is urgently needed to confirm or rule out relationships between disorganized feeding and birth practices, events, and interventions.

Summary Points for Protecting the Mother-Baby Continuum

- The infant's ability to suck, swallow, and breathe during feeding is controlled by 6 cranial nerves and some 60 muscles, acting on 22 bones in the infant skull.
- Muscles in the infant mouth function best when hydrated and nourished, and may be injured or mispatterned during and shortly after childbirth.
- Mechanical forces during birth can disrupt the alignment of bony structures and therefore affect nerve and muscle function.
- Instrument-assisted birth and cesarean birth exert additional mechanical forces on bony structures in the infant over and above the levels of force during spontaneous vaginal birth.
- Assuring adequate hydration and caloric support for the infant and establishing and maintaining the mother's milk supply are necessities in the interim. This should occur in the context of a supportive mother-infant relationship.

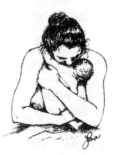

References

1. Cregan MD, Hartmann PE. 1999. Computerized breast measurement from conception to weaning: Clinical implications. *J Hum Lact* 15(2):89–96.
2. Woolridge, M. Anatomy of infant sucking. 1986. *Midwifery* 2:164–171.
3. Halpern SH, Levine T, Wilson DB, et al. 1999. Effect of labor analgesia on breastfeeding success. *Birth* 26(2):83–88.
4. Soskolne EI, Schumacher R, Fyock C, et al. 1996. The effect of early discharge and other factors on readmission rates of newborns. *Arch Pediatr Adolesc Med* 150(4):373–379.

5. Edmonson MB, Stoddard JJ, Owens LM. 1997. Hospital readmission with feeding-related problems after early postpartum discharge of normal newborns. *JAMA* 378(4):299–303.
6. Bertini G, Dani C, Tronchin M, Rubaltelli FF. 2001. Is breastfeeding really favoring early neonatal jaundice? *Pediatrics* 107(3). *www.pediatrics.org/cgi/content/full/1073/e41*
7. Montagu A. 1986. *Touching: The Human Significance of the Skin,* 3rd ed. New York: Harper and Row, 1986.
8. Hrdy, SB. 1999. *Mother Nature: A History of Mothers, Infants, and Natural Selection.* New York: Pantheon Books.
9. Tuchman DN, Walter RS. 1994. *Disorders of Feeding and Swallowing in Infants and Children: Pathophysiology, Diagnosis and Treatment.* San Diego: Singuar Publishing Group, Inc.
10. Netter FH. *Atlas of Human Anatomy.* Summit, NJ: CIBA-Geigy Corporation, 1989.
11. Wolf LS, Glass RP. 1992. *Feeding and Swallowing Disorders in Infancy: Assessment and Management.* Tucson, AZ: Therapy Skill Builders/Communicator Skills Builders.
12. Arvedson JC, Brodsky L. 1993. *Pediatric swallowing and feeding: Assessment and management.* San Diego, CA: Singular Publishing Group.
13. Palmer MM, Crawley K, Blanco IA. Neonatal oral-motor assessment scale: A reliability study. *J Perinato* 8(1):28–35.
14. Daly SE, Di Rosso A, Owens RA, Hartmann PE. 1993. Degree of breast emptying explains changes in the fat content, but not fatty acid composition, of human milk. *Exp Physiol.* 78(6):741–55.
15. Daly SEJ, Kent JC, Huynh DQ, et al. 1996. The determination of short-term volume changes and the rate of synthesis of human milk using computerized breast measurement. *Exper Physiol* 77:79–87.
16. Ward RC, ed. 2003. *Foundations for Osteopathic Medicine,* 2nd ed. Philadelphia: Lippincott Williams and Wilkins.
17. Csontos F, Rush M, Hollt V, et al. 1979. Elevated plasma beth-endorphin levels in pregnant women and their neonates. *Life Sci* 25:835–844.
18. Vermes I, Kaitar I, Szabo F. 1979. Changes of maternal and fetal pituitary-adrenocorticals functions during human labor. *Horm Res* 11:213–217.
19. Li CH, Yumashiro D, Tsent LF, et al. 1977. Synthesis and analgesic activity of human beta-endorphin. *J Med Chem* 29:325–328.
20. Gray L, Miller LW, Philipp BI, et al. 2002. Breastfeeding is analgesic in healthy newborns. *Pediatrics* 109:590–593.
21. Zanardo V, Nicolussi S, Giacomin C, et al. 2001. Labor pain effects on colostral milk beta-endorphin concentrations of lactating mothers. *Biol Neonate* 79:87–90.
22. Fryman VM. Relation of disturbances of craniosacral mechanism to symptomatology of the newborn: Study of 1250 infants. *J Am Osteo Assoc* 65:1059–1075.

23. Fryman VM. 1998. Cerebral dysfunction: Prevention and treatment in the light of the osteopathic concept. In *The Collected Papers of Viola M. Fryman, DO: Legacy of Osteopathy to Children.* Indianapolis, IN: American Academy of Osteopathy.

24. Peitsch WK, Keefer CH, LaBrie RA, et al. 2002. Incidence of cranial asymmetry in healthy newborns. *Pediatrics* 110(6):72. *www.pediatrics.org/cgi/content/full/110/6/37*

25. Woolridge M. 1986. Aetiology of sore nipples. *Midwifery* 2:172–176.

26. Korones SB. 1976. *High-risk Newborn Infants.* 2nd ed. St. Louis: CV Mosby.

27. Amiel-Tison C, Sureau C, Shnider SM. Cerebral Handicap in full-term neonates related to the mechanical forces of labor. 1988. *Bailleres Clin Obstet Gynaecol* 2(1):145–165.

28. Hall RT, Mercer AM, Teasley SL, et al. 2002. A breastfeeding assessment score to evaluate the risk for cessation of breastfeeding by 7 to 10 days of age. *J Ped* 141:659–664.

29. FDA Public Health Advisory: *Need for CAUTION When Using Vacuum Assisted Delivery Devices.* Washington DC: Food and Drug Administration, May 21, 1998. *http://www.fda.gov/cdrh/fetal598.html*

30. Tappero EP, Honeyfield ME. 1993. *Physical Assessment of the Newborn.* Petaluma, CA: NICULink Book Publishers.

31. Blair A. 2001. *Sore Nipples and Breastfeeding: Assessment of the Relationship Between Positioning and Pain.* School of Interdisciplinary Arts and Sciences. Cincinnati, Union Institute and University.

32. Smith WL, Erenberg A, Nowak, A. 1988. Imaging evaluation of the human nipple during breastfeeding. *Am J Dis Child* 142: 76–78.

33. Black LS. Baby-Friendly Newborn Care. Workshop for Lactation Specialists, Series VIII. Chicago: La Leche League International, 1993.

34. Boshart CA. 2001. *The Pacifier: Making the Decision.* Temecula, CA: Speech Dynamics Inc.

35. Caton D, Frolich MA, Euliano TY. 2002. Anesthesia for childbirth: Controversy and change. In "The nature and management of labor pain: Peer-reviewed papers from an evidence-based symposium. *Suppl Am J Obstetrics Gynecol* May 2002: S25–S30.

36. Loftus J, Hill H, Cohen S. 1995. Placental transfer and neonatal effects of epidural sufentanil and fentanyl administered with bupivicaine during labor. *Anesthesiol,* 83:300–308.

37. Baumgarder DJ, Muehl P, Fischer M, Pribbenow B. 2003. Effect of labor epidural anesthesia on breastfeeding of healthy full-term newborns delivered vaginally. *J Am Board Fam Pract* 16(1):7–13.

38. Rooks J, Sakala C, Corey M. The Nature and Management of Labor Pain: Peer-reviewd papers from an evidence-based symposium. *Suppl Am J Obstet Gynecol* May 2002:186(5).
39. Powers NG. 2002. Dealing with infant problems during breastfeeding. Presentation to Pediatrix Medical Group of Kansas, Wesley Medical Center, Wichita, KS.
40. World Health Organization. 1998. *Evidence for the Ten Steps to Successful Breastfeeding.* Geneva: World Health Organization WHO/CHD/98.9.
41. Christensson K, Cabrera T, Christensson E, et al. 1995. Separation distress call in the human neonate in the absence of maternal body contact. *Acta Paediatr* 84(5):468–473.
42. Anderson GC. 1989. Risk in mother-infant separation postbirth. *Image* 21(4):196–199.
43. Avrahami E, Amzel S, Katz R, et al. 1996. CT demonstration of intracranial bleeding in term newborns with mild clinical symptoms. *Clin Radiol* 51:31–34.
44. Carbajal R, Veerapen S, Couderc S, et al. 2003. Analgesic effect of breastfeeding in term neonates: Randomized controlled trial. *Brit Med J* 326(7379):13–15.
45. Daly SEJ, and Hartmann, PE. 1995. Infant demand and milk supply. Part 1: Infant demand and milk supply in lactating women. *J Hum Lact* 11:21–26.
    Daly SEJ, and Hartmann, PE. 1995. Infant demand and milk supply. Part 2: The short-term control of milk synthesis in lactating women. *J Hum Lact* 11:27–31.
46. Labbok MH, and Hendershot GE. 1987. Does breastfeeding protect against malocclusion? An analysis of the 1981 child health supplement to the National Health Interview Survey. *Am J Prev Med* 3(4):227–232.
47. Owens J, Opipari L, Nobile C, et al. 1998. Sleep and daytime behavior in children with obstructive sleep apnea and behavioral sleep disorders. *Pediatrics* 102(5):1178.
48. Locklin, Maryanne. "When Breastfeeding does not work: the emotional impact." Presentation at the 8th Annual Conference for Advanced Practitioners, Rush University, Chicago, March 22, 2001.
49. Fraval M. 1998. A pilot study: Osteopathic treatment of infants with a sucking dysfunction. *J Am Acad Ost* 8(2):25–33.
50. O'Connell JA, McCarroll CJ, Smith LJ, et al. 1993. Effects of osteopathic manipulative therapy on suck disorders in the newborn. Dayton, OH: Proposal to National Institutes of Health Exploratory Grants for Alternative Medicine, June 1993.

CHAPTER 8

EPISIOTOMY AND SURGICAL DELIVERY AND BREASTFEEDING

"Episiotomy fits with the obstetric premise that childbirth is a dangerous and difficult business and that the obstetrician's role is to rescue the baby."

Henci Goer, Author, 1999

Episiotomy: Background Information

Episiotomy, the surgical incision of a woman's perineum to enlarge the vagina at delivery, is the most common obstetrical operation in the world, excluding cutting of the umbilical cord. In the United States, episiotomy is the most common type of incision made on any female.[1] When natural childbirth activists were questioning why 70–80% of all North American births involved routine use of episiotomy, Kitzenger wrote, "this is the only surgical intervention which takes place on the body of a healthy woman without her consent and often without informing her."[2]

As discussed in Chapter 4, episiotomy was introduced in the United States in 1920s when use of the lithotomy position and sedation at delivery were becoming common practice in hospitals.[3] That this operation persists in spite of the fact that research does not support its routine use is another example of obstetrical "culture lag" because only evidence-based practices are used.

Scientific Literature has Questioned Episiotomy for Decades

Over twenty years ago, a comprehensive review of the English language literature on episiotomy was conducted by the Center for Disease Control.[4] Some 350 articles and chapters from books were reviewed, dating from 1860–1980. Their methodology allowed for inclusion of many studies that would be disqualified as nonscientific, but they rekindled the dialogue on this practice. Their review cited three major "medical" justifications given for episiotomy:

- Prevention of third-degree laceration of the perineum
- Prevention of serious damage to the pelvic wall
- Prevention of trauma to the infant head

Also covered were the documented risks of episiotomy, including extension to a deeper tear, unsatisfactory anatomic results, blood loss, pain and swelling, and infection. The lengthy paper concludes that "arguments for widespread use of episiotomy do not withstand scientific scrutiny...and the risks of episiotomy have been largely ignored."

Since this review, findings of several more studies support no physiologic advantage to mothers or infants in uncomplicated deliveries, and one study cited better perineal healing among women without episiotomies compared to those who had them.[5–7]

In 1992, a large, randomized, controlled clinical trial in Canada studied 675 healthy mothers at term who had been randomized into two groups, one with restrictive episiotomy use and one with liberal (hospital routine) use of episiotomy. The method of management of the perineum at delivery was directed by random assignment of the birth attendant to either "try to avoid episiotomy" for the experimental group or "try to avoid a tear" for the control group. Results confirmed that restriction of episiotomy resulted in significantly more women having intact perineum and need for less suturing. Multiparous women in the "restricted" episiotomy group more often gave birth with intact perineum, and women in all groups who gave birth with an intact perineum "fared best" in terms of immediate postpartum pain and pelvic floor relaxation, as well as pain and vaginal tone at three months post delivery. Additionally, routine use of median episiotomy was associated with more third- and fourth-degree lacerations. Overall, these authors concluded that there was no evidence for liberal or routine use of episiotomy.

More "Culture Lag"?

A large epidemiological study in 18 large urban hospitals in the United States quantified episiotomy rates in nulliparas women during a two-month period in 1994.[8] During that period, 49,692 spontaneous vaginal deliveries occurred in study hospitals with

16,722 (34%) being to first-time mothers who are considered at greatest risk for perineal trauma at birth. Mothers with confounding risk factors were eliminated, and the final sample was 14,292 (85% of all nulliparas). Results showed that episiotomy rates among the 18 hospitals were high, ranging from 20% to 73% of deliveries. Third- and fourth-degree lacerations were statistically corrected to episiotomy. These authors conclude that the continued high use of episiotomy, citing a rate of over 20% in any hospital as being too high, reflects a trend consistent with findings in clinical trials and they argue that "liberal use of episiotomy is unwarranted and probably even harmful." These findings are corroborated in the National Maternity Center Survey, which reported 27% episiotomy rate among its respondents.[9]

Episiotomy in Developing Countries and Resource-Poor Settings

What about episiotomy use in developing countries? An editorial in the *British Medical Journal* entitled "Routine Episiotomy in Developing Countries: Time to Change a Harmful Practice," reports on a 1998 "straw poll" on episiotomy use of midwives from five African countries and Nepal, who were attending courses in Liverpool.[10] Although this was a small, nonrandom sample, participants at international courses are often from senior positions and are likely to know national statistics. Most respondents indicated that episiotomy is still a routine on all primagravidas in their countries (see Figure 8-1). The author of the study followed-up with a Medline search that revealed little additional quantitative data. Studies are cited from Burkina Faso, which reported 43% of all first-time mothers having episiotomy and from Botswana, which reported 1 in every 3 mothers delivering normally has an episiotomy.

In a developing country context, one of the greatest concerns for episiotomy complications and long-term maternal morbidity is the risk of "dehiscence" (breaking down) of a repair and ensuing rectovaginal fistula (literally a hole between the vagina and rectum whereby feces pass out the vaginal opening). A comprehensive review of obstetrical literature in the English language was done in 1994, with articles dating back as far as the 1930s analyzed for episiotomy and sequelae.[11] The authors conclude that episiotomy brings a strong risk for extension into the rectum and persistent rectovaginal fistula. In many very traditional cultures, with religious or other taboos against feces, a chronic fistula could be cause for a woman's ostracism from her family or even divorce.

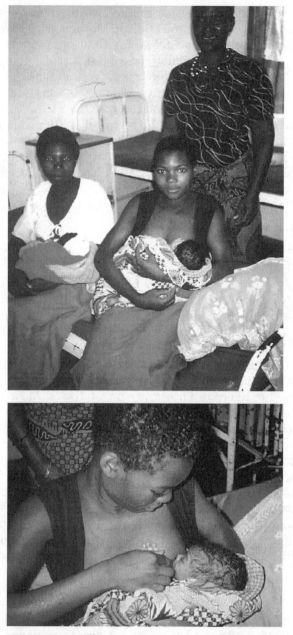

FIGURE 8-1 All primiparas in this rural hospital in Malawi are delivered with episiotomy. This young mother, 17 years old, had difficulty finding a comfortable way to sit and breastfeed her baby because of the incision pain. Virtually all mothers breastfeed in Malawi and assistance with difficulties is provided by her mother. *Photo by Mary Kroeger, 2001.*

Episiotomy and Breastfeeding

Does episiotomy pain affect early breastfeeding success? If pain and the accompanying tension and anxiety inhibit oxytocin release, then marked perineal discomfort could be a factor influencing breastfeeding. Kitzinger conducted a large retrospective qualitative study in England on women's perception of their episiotomy pain.[12] Included in the questionnaire were questions on whether the women's perineal pain had distracted them while breastfeeding or if they could sit comfortably while holding their baby. Many respondents said they forgot about their pain when feeding their babies, but 17% of the episiotomy group and 21% of those who had episiotomies with lacerations were "troubled by perineal pain a lot, often, or always" while feeding, compared to 3% of women who had no injury to the perineum. In addition, 68% of the mothers with episiotomies reported that they had to be careful when sitting and, of these, 18% said they sat with difficulty (see Table 8-1).

WHO has taken a stand that episiotomy should not be routine.[13-15] The publication *Managing Complications in Pregnancy and Childbirth: A Guide for Midwives and Doctors*, which gives guidelines for obstetrical care in developing country settings, states:

> Episiotomy is no longer recommended as a routine procedure. There is no evidence that routine episiotomy decreases perineal damage, future vaginal prolapse or urinary incontinence. In fact routine episiotomy is associated with an increase in third and fourth degree tears and subsequent anal sphincter muscle dysfunction.

TABLE 8-1   Pain in Perineum Distracted Woman When Breastfeeding

	Not at all	A bit/ occasionally	A lot, often, always	Total
Tear	234 (68%)	79 (23%)	31 (9%)	344
Episiotomy	409 (43%)	381 (40%)	167 (17%)	957
Episiotomy & Tear	55 (37%)	62 (42%)	31 (21%)	148
Intact	154 (92%)	9 (5%)	5 (3%)	168
Total	852 (53%)	531 (33%)	234 (14%)	1617

From Kitzinger S., 1981. Reprinted with permission.[12]

Episiotomy Interferes with Early Initiation

Besides being a painful and possibly damaging and disfiguring procedure for the mother, episiotomy repair can influence bonding, skin-to-skin care, and early initiation of breastfeeding. If a mother needs stitches, the nurse usually takes the baby during the repair thinking that the mother may drop the baby while she remains (or is put) in lithotomy position for repair. In U.S. hospitals, babies are put on radiant warmers during the suturing and many newborn admitting procedures may be performed, including cord care, eye drop instillation, weighing, measuring, and even bathing the baby. Many of these procedures have been shown to interfere with early effective breastfeeding.[16] In resource-poor settings babies may simply be put on a side table without any radiant warming device and these babies can and do get cold. Although many delivery tables are far from optimal for skin-to-skin contact and early initiation, reordering nursing priorities can bring the nurse to the bedside to support the mother who is being sutured. These early moments are the most important for the mother-baby dyad, and all other routines should be set aside to help that mother to meet and hold her baby (see Chapter 10). Appropriate anesthesics must be administered to reduce the pain of suturing, and a nurse, labor companion, relative, or maternity staff member should stay at the mother's side. Midwifery refresher training has shown that maternity care providers can change their routines (see Figure 8-2).

Moyses Paciornik, whose video about birth in the squatting position was discussed in Chapter 4, has written about his expe-

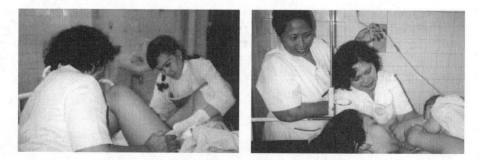

FIGURE 8-2 Midwifery refresher training in Indonesia introduced the "new" practice of putting the baby skin-to-skin on mother immediately after delivery. This not only supports early breastfeeding, but also distracts the mother who looks at and touches her newborn. Nurse-midwives stayed nearby for support and assistance. *Photo by Mary Kroeger, ACNM LSS © Training, Jakarta, 1996.*

rience. In a decade of work with over 14,000 deliveries by "civilized women" in the squatting position, he has learned that episiotomy is never indicated.[17] The majority (70%) of the women he observed/attended sustained no laceration or very small tears. He argues that in the upright squat position, all the anatomic and physiologic forces work optimally and, with the mother herself in control of the delivery (as the film depicts), large tears are uncommon. He also reinforces the empowerment a mother apparently feels in this position, and he reinforces the connection between the peace and control this position imparts to the mother and her readiness to touch, cuddle, and breastfeed her infant.

Cesarean Section: Background Information

A cesarean section (CS), or surgical delivery of a baby through the mother's abdomen, can be a life-saving intervention for mother, fetus, or both. Based on global data, WHO estimates that the CS rate should not exceed 10–15%, even in a high-risk referral facility.[18,19] Cesarean rates are on the rise in many parts of the world and have reached shocking numbers in some countries. In the last thirty years, CS rates in the United States rose sharply, climbing from 4.5% of all births in 1965 to 16.5% in 1980, and jumping again to 24.7% in 1988. The rates declined slightly in the early 1990s as more women sought vaginal birth after a primary C-section (VBAC), but the rates began to climb again, and in 2001 the rate was back to 24.5% of all births (Figure 8-3). One explanation for the CS rate turning upwards again is that fewer VBACs are being attempted. VBAC has long been common in Europe (where it is termed "trial of scar"), in Africa, and in most resource-poor countries.[20]

Box 8-1   CS and VBAC Rates: A Marker of the Move away from Vaginal Delivery?

In the United States, the practice of VBAC began to increase when a national effort to reduce the CS rate was undertaken.[21] Between 1990 and 2000, the VBAC rates increased and peaked at 36% of all mothers with previous CS, and then began to drop again because of limited evidence that there is additional risk of complications (See Figure 8-3).[23] The *ACOG Bulletin*

continued

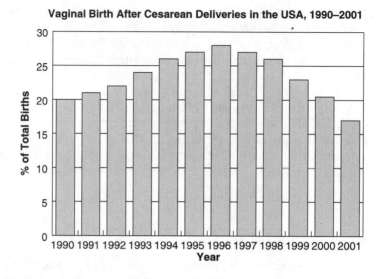

Vaginal Birth After Cesarean Deliveries in the USA, 1990–2001

FIGURE 8-3 US VBAC Rates, 1990–2001[22]

Box 8-1 continued

released in 1999 set forth new recommendations that "VBAC should only be attempted in institutions equipped to respond to emergencies with physicians immediately available."[24] This recommendation is not based on compelling evidence, yet it is having a major impact on childbirth choices in small and community maternity hospitals nationwide where obstetricians, anesthesiologists, and other surgical staff are on call from home.

For example, the rural practice in Kauai, Hawaii, where the author previously worked with a busy obstetrician-nurse-midwife collaborative practice, saw a drop in their VBAC rate from 32.8% in 1999, to 24% in 2000, to 13.4% in 2001. In March 2002, VBAC was stopped at this island altogether due to the hospital's decision to follow the ACOG recommendations. The hospital did not have the resources to pay surgical staff to stay "in-house" 24 hours a day. Thus, all mothers with previous CS are now delivered by repeat CS, or they have to fly (at their own expense) to the Island of Oahu for a VBAC. Reports from a childbirth educator/lactation consultant there are that essentially all previous cesarean section mothers stay and have the CS.[25]

In the United Kingdom the CS rates are also rising, with the rate in 1997 nearing 20% of all deliveries (30% in some hospitals), compared to 10% in 1990—the rate doubled in a decade.[26,27,28] There is a simultaneous trend towards increasing births with medications, particularly epidural anesthesic.[27]

Latin America, Argentina, Brazil, and Paraguay have national CS rates exceeding 40%, and in Chile, Colombia, and Mexico, rates exceed 50%.[29] CS rates are higher in private hospitals, but even public-sector facilities have rates far higher than the 10-15% recommended by the WHO. Based on these data, the 12 Latin American countries having CS rates above 15% are countries that account for 81% of all births in the region. This means many mother-infant pairs are affected.

Chile has the highest CS rate in the world. A Chilean midwife has reviewed the literature to find the reasons given for the high CS rate in her country. These reasons include the traditionally accepted clinical factors like fetal distress, cephalopelvic disproportion, breech and other mal-presentation, and previous c-section, along with failed induction of labor, obesity, and high maternal age.[30] The non-medical factors include, socioeconomic status (higher income women use private hospitals and are more likely to have a C-section), educational level, type of insurance held, type of training the physician had, fear of litigation, scheduling for convenience of mother or doctor, women's fear of the pain of labor, and finally, knowledge that vaginal birth causes pelvic floor damage. Very few of these indications would have been considered valid indications thirty years ago in any country. Women and families are not being made fully aware of the risk of the surgery to themselves, their baby, and to breastfeeding.

This trend is not confined to Latin America. In Thailand, according to 2000 data, CS rates were 24%, 48%, and 22% for general, private, and university hospitals, respectively.[31] In Shanghai, China, over the last three decades, CS rates have increased from 4.7% to 22.5%.[32] The Chinese study found that the dramatic rise in surgical delivery was due less to "the factors that usually lead to cesarean sections" and more to emerging health insurance and fee-for-service payments.

This apparent link between CS rates and a population's ability to pay for this procedure is most apparent in resource poor Africa. There, where the CS rates have always been very low, CS rates are now seen to be dropping in many countries.[30] For example, in Zambia, where more than 20% of all pregnant mothers are HIV-infected, there has been a drop in CS rates in the past decade from close to 3% of all births to less than 2%. This trend in Africa is of particular irony, as in the United States and Europe, women-who are HIV positive have elective CS as the standard of care to reduce risks of HIV transmission to the baby.

The rising CS rate in the urban centers of both developed and developing countries is changing the global attitude about child-birth. The "convenience" of the cesarean birth is an idea being exported in a way similar to the export of bottle-feeding decades ago. There can be little doubt that there is a similar profit motive in this trend.

Cesarean Section is Major Abdominal Surgery

Cesarean delivery is a major surgical intervention that encom-passes many different interventions and thus presents a particu-lar challenge for studying its impact on breastfeeding. A woman undergoing CS will at the least have her belly prepped and shaved, most of her body covered with sterile drapes, a urinary catheter placed, IVs started, monitors of her vital signs and the fetal vital signs attached—all of this in a generally cold and very bright room. Even with a planned CS, these interventions can be fright-ening to anyone. If the CS is an emergency, due to life-threaten-ing events for fetus or mother, fear of harm or death for herself or her baby will be added to the unfamiliar events that are unfold-ing. The CS may follow what was already a long, difficult labor that included many of the interventions already discussed in con-nection with breastfeeding outcomes: confinement to bed, fasting, analgesia and/or anesthesics for pain, oxytocin augmentation, and anxiety and stress. In many countries, mothers are not allowed a supportive companion to be present for the delivery. Anesthesics and other medications will be administered.

The baby born by CS has more respiratory problems at birth, because the baby does not descend through the vaginal outlet to delivery and thus misses out on hormonal and physical stresses, not fully understood, but which are believed to bring the baby to extra-uterine life ready to feed. These physiologic effects of the delivery on the baby will be discussed further in Chapters 9 and 10. CS-born babies are often born with considerable mucous and need additional suctioning of mouth and throat, also risk factors for successful breastfeeding (see Chapter 7).

Postpartum, a mother delivered by CS starts her new relation-ship with her baby in less than optimal terms. Even when regional anesthesic rather than general anesthesic has been used and where the maternity staff is committed to the earliest possible initiation of breastfeeding, there will be some delay. Until the Baby Friendly

(BFHI) principles, or "Ten Steps to Successful Breastfeeding," became the standards of care, most infants of CS-delivered mothers received one or several supplemental feedings before the first breastfeed. Infants of CS mothers still frequently remain in the nursery, rather than rooming-in, until the mother can get up and move around. The new mother will have to cope with incision pain from major abdominal surgery and with lingering side effects of anesthesia. She may have complications of infection, pneumonia, and a nicked bladder or intestine. Sometimes she will have a sense of failure or depression about her inability to deliver normally.

Cesarean section is riskier than vaginal birth, and even in industrialized countries maternal mortality is two times higher with CS as compared to vaginal delivery. In settings where staffing is inadequate, infection prevention is often not rigorous, and antibiotics are not always available, complications of CS still are a significant cause of maternal mortality and morbidity.[32-34]

Literature Reviews on Cesarean Section and Breastfeeding

Given this backdrop, the research on the impact of CS on breastfeeding success is difficult to sort out, and many findings are conflicting. Study design and outcome variables are often very different and it is hard to compare findings. Several studies point to cesarean delivery as having a negative impact on breastfeeding success, particularly during the early postpartum period.[35-37] However, two of these studies cite separation between mother and infant for up to 12 hours and early supplementation with formula as major confounding factors. In the third study, the mothers in the cesarean group supplemented their babies with formula and fed less at night. All three studies also looked at CS and its impact on duration of breastfeeding. The Samuels study reports that CS mothers were more likely to stop breastfeeding within the first 2 weeks postpartum than mothers who delivered vaginally. Procianoy found that CS mothers were significantly less likely to be breastfeeding at 2 months than mothers who had vaginal births. The Vestermark study found that breastfeeding mothers in the CS group had a later onset of full lactation during the first four days postpartum, but of those mothers who were breastfeeding at discharge, there was no statistical difference at 3 and 6 months among the three methods of delivery studied: vaginal, vacuum extraction, and CS.

A prospective study found no difference in breastfeeding outcomes by delivery method. The study of 215 postpartum mothers in an Alaskan hospital with a 28% CS rate investigated mode of delivery and other factors associated with breastfeeding success.[39] Mothers were interviewed in the hospital and then again at 6 weeks postpartum. Findings were that there was no statistical difference in breastfeeding rates at six weeks postpartum among vaginally delivered mothers compared to those delivered by cesarean section. The author, Janke, a nurse-researcher, found that "commitment to breastfeeding" was associated with breastfeeding success regardless of mode of delivery, and that among the CS mothers, it was the only variable associated with success. This is an important finding since good support and motivation have been recognized as key indicators of breastfeeding success. A motivated, experienced mother who has a scheduled repeat C-section may have little trouble initiating breastfeeding. A primigravida who has an emergency CS for fetal distress after a long, difficult labor is in a qualitatively different situation. Motivation and close support would be a critical factor for this latter mother.

Another finding on factors affecting breastfeeding in mothers who have had CS is the impact of early suckling. In a prospective study done in 1992 in Turkey, 40 mothers of healthy term babies born by CS under general anesthesia were randomly divided into two groups.[40] In Turkey, as in much of the developing world, CS is still done under general anesthesia and mothers take longer to recover from anesthesia and become awake enough to hold and breastfeed their infants. Twenty mothers were assisted in suckling their babies at one hour after birth and then assisted to feed frequently thereafter. In the control group, 20 babies of CS-delivered mothers were supplemented first with glucose water and not put to breast until a mean time of 20 hours after delivery, the earliest being 6 hours after delivery. In the early breastfed group, mothers were able to express colostrum on the average at 8.3 hours (range 5–12 hours) after delivery. In the control group, colostrum was not expressed until 33.6 hours after delivery (range 10–60 hours). Let-down sensation by 12–30 hours after delivery was noted by the mothers in the early suckling group, compared to 36–60 hours in the controls. These authors conclude that early suckling after CS delivery promotes significantly earlier colostrum and breast milk secretion.

The possible direct effect of cesarean delivery on the infant has been investigated with attention to the level of circulating catecholamines in umbilical plasma samples. A group in Sweden looked at 30 full-term infants, half born by elective cesarean section and half born vaginally.[41] Infants born after CS were less excitable and had significantly decreased neurological responses during the first two days post delivery. When umbilical plasma samples taken from each infant at delivery were analyzed, the mean catecholamine concentrations were significantly lower in the cesarean-born infants. These authors hypothesize that the higher catecholamine surge at the moment of vaginal delivery may be of importance in the early neurological responses in the newborn. More research in this area is needed.

In another study by a different group at the same Swedish institution, hormonal patterns were compared in 20 woman delivered vaginally and in 17 mothers delivered by emergency CS.[42] On day 2 after delivery, all mothers were blood sampled for oxytocin, prolactin, and cortisol. Mothers were also given a standardized personality test on the third day postpartum to assess anxiety levels and were followed up at 2 months postpartum with another questionnaire that documented the length of time they had exclusively breastfed. The vaginally delivered mothers had significantly more oxytocin pulses than the CS mothers and also had significant rises in prolactin levels at 20–30 minutes after onset of breastfeeding. The number of pulses was correlated to duration of exclusive breastfeeding in the vaginal delivery group. This study is complex and the authors' discussion suggests a possible relationship between oxytocin pulsations and early prolactin secretion. A key finding is that vaginal delivery seems to foster earlier, more effective secretion of the two key hormones associated with lactation.

A prospective longitudinal study in Australia published in 2002 looked specifically at the impact of operative delivery on implementation of Step Four of the Baby Friendly Hospital Initiative (BFHI), "early initiation of breastfeeding within 30 minutes of birth." (The Australia Baby Friendly criteria say within 60 minutes of birth, and this is the criterion used in the study.)[43] Before delivery, a representative sociodemographic sample of 203 primiparas was enlisted. They were all planning to deliver at one of four hospitals, only one of which was a Baby Friendly hospital. The mothers were visited in the hospital at 2 days postpartum and again 8 months after delivery. Cross-checking hospital records corroborated delivery information. Findings were that mothers who had delivered by cesarean section had significant delays in early breastfeeding. This delay was significantly longer in the three non-BFHI hospitals compared to vaginal birth whether spontaneous or assisted. They also found that of the mothers who delivered by CS at the BFHI hospital, 27% had initiated breastfeeding by 30 minutes after delivery and 60% by 60 minutes. In the three non-BFHI hospitals, none of the mothers surgically delivered had put her baby to breast. These findings are consistent with the findings of Janke that a climate of support and intent to breastfeed works positively for all mothers, regardless of mode of delivery.

Conclusions

The escalating CS rate in the United States, Europe, Latin America, and parts of Asia should be noted with great concern by all maternity care providers, including lactation care providers. It is a "marker" for measuring the increasing medicalization of maternity care as a whole. Obstetricians are themselves "opting" for elective CS and this trend gives a powerful message to their patients.[33,34] In spite of scholarly journals, popular magazine and newspaper articles, books, pamphlets, videos, radio and TV programs, professional meetings and conferences, and most significantly, in spite of standards and guidelines set by global policy makers like WHO, the "birth machine," as Wagner has called it, seems to be rolling on down the road to the future.[45]

Discussion in depth of the cultural, economic, and political reasons for the climbing global CS rate is beyond the scope of this book. However, postpartum care providers need to know the impact of these medicalized labors and surgical births on mothers and babies. The unethical marketing and promotion of breastmilk substitutes to both mothers and health care providers that was exposed in the 1970s and finally regulated by the *International Code of Marketing Breast-milk Substitutes*[46] has its worrying parallel in medical technology. This marketing approach is not a new phenomenon to breastfeeding activists. Pharmaceutical companies and medical equipment vendors visit obstetrical practices and maternity hospitals regularly. Pens, note pads, and other items with the logo of certain brands of labor analgesics or anesthetics come with free samples of other medications for health providers. The vendors of electronic fetal monitors, vacuum extractors, and other obstetrical technical equipment host medical in-service education meetings. Medical equipment and pharmaceutical companies are just as aware now of the profit to be gained by a globally increasing surgical delivery rate as was the baby food industry decades ago.

The issue is further clouded by the call for the "women's right to choose." In much the same way there have been advocates for the "right" not to breastfeed, there are advocates for free choice of anesthesia in labor or choice of an elective cesarean section. A woman also has a right to know all the possible long-term and short-term side effects of medications and obstetrical procedures, just as a mother who chooses to formula feed her newborn needs to be well educated about the reasons why breastfeeding is the best way to feed her newborn.

The global breastfeeding community must first see the clear links between childbirth and breastfeeding. Breastfeeding as the norm for most mothers in the 21st century is a goal we are far from reaching, and medicalized birth, particularly the rising CS rates in so many settings, threatens to make this goal even harder to attain.

Summary Points for Protecting the Mother-Baby Continuum

- Episiotomy is no longer recommended as a routine obstetric procedure and there is no evidence that it decreases perineal damage and other reproductive tract complications.
- Mothers with no or minimal perineal trauma will be more comfortable and relaxed breastfeeding in the first hours and days of life.
- Cesarean sections are life saving when used appropriately, but they are being performed in inappropriately high numbers in some settings and nations.
- Evidence linking CS to breastfeeding difficulty is conflicting; however, some well-designed studies show a clear link between CS and later initiation of and shorter duration of breastfeeding.
- Evidence shows that an infant and mother from a CS delivery requires greater support to ensure breastfeeding success and that motivation is an important variable.
- Evidence suggests that vaginal delivery fosters earlier, more effective secretion of two key hormones associated with lactation than delivery by CS.

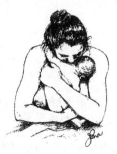

References

1. Popovic JR. 1999. *National Hospital Discharge Survey: Annual Summary with Detailed Diagnosis and Procedure Data.* Vital and Health Statistics Series 13 no. 151. Hyattsville, MD: National Center for Health Statistics.
2. Kitzinger S. 1981. Pamphlet. *Some Women's Experiences of Episiotomy.* London: The National Childbirth Trust, NLM # 05304054-6.
3. DeLee JB. 1920. The prophylactic forceps operation. *Am J Obstet Gynecol,* 1:34–44.
4. Thacker SB, Banta HD. 1983. Benefits and risks of episiotomy: An interpretive review of the English language literature, 1960-1980. *Obstet Gynecol Survey,* 38:322–338.
5. Harrison RF, Brennen M, North PM, et al. 1984. Is routine episiotomy necessary? *Br Med J,* 288:1971–1975.
6. Formato L. 1985. Routine prophylactic episiotomy: Is it always necessary? *J Nurse Midwif,* 30(3):144–148.
7. McGuinness M, Norr K, Nacion K. 1985. Comparison between different perineal outcomes on tissue healing. *J Nurse Midwif,* 36(3):192–198.
8. Webb DA, Culhane J. 2002. Hospital variation in episiotomy use and the risk of perineal trauma during childbirth. *Birth,* 29(2):132–137.
9. Declercq ER, Sakala C, Corry MP, et al. 2002. *Listening to Mothers: Report of the First National U.S. Survey of Women's Childbearing Experiences.* New York: Maternity Center Association October 2002. *www.maternity.org/listeningto mothers/results.html.*
10. Maduma-Butshe A. 1998. Routine episiotomy in developing countries: Time to change a harmful practice. *BMJ,* 316:1179–1180.
11. Homsi R, Daikoku NH, Littlejohn J, et al. 1994. Episiotomy: Risks of dehiscence and rectovaginal fistula. *Obstet Gynecol Survey,* 49(12):803–808.
12. Kitzinger S. 1981. Pamphlet: *Some Women's Experiences of Episiotomy.* London: The National Childbirth Trust, NLM # 05304054-6.
13. Thompson A. 1997. Episiotomies should not be routine. *Safe Motherhood Newsletter,* 12. WHO, Geneva.
14. WHO, UNFPA, UNICEF, World Bank. 2000. *Managing Complications in Pregnancy and Childbirth: A Guide for Midwives and Doctors.* World Health Organization. Department of Reproductive Health and Research, C-59.
15. Chalmers B, Mangiaterra V, Porter R. 2001. WHO principles of perinatal care: The essential antenatal, perinatal, and postnatal care course. *Birth,* 28(3):202–207.

16. Righard L, Alade MO. 1990. Effect of delivery room routines on success of first breast-feed. *Lancet*, 336:1105–1107.

17. Paciornik M.1990. Commentary: Arguments against episiotomy and in favor of squatting for birth. *Birth*, 17(2):104–105.

18. WHO. 1985. Appropriate technology for birth. *Lancet*, 2:436–437.

19. Wagner M.1993. An epidemic of unnecessary cesareans. *Mothering*, Fall:71–73.

20. Flamm BL. 2001. Vaginal birth after cesarean (VBAC). *Best Pract Res Clin Obstet Gynaecol* 15(1):81–92.

21. Department of Health and Human Services. 1991. *Healthy People 2000: National Promotion and Disease Prevention Objectives.* Washington, DC: US Department of Health and Human Services. Publication # HRSA-M-CH-91-92.

22. Data for graph from: NCHS Hospital Discharge Surveys *www.cdc.gov/nchs*. Pubs under Birth 2002 US VBAC Rates, 1990–2001.

23. Goer H. 2002. The assault on normal birth: The OB disinformation campaign. *Midwifery Today*, 63:10–14.

24. ACOG Practice Bulletin #5. July 1999. *Vaginal birth after previous cesarean section*. American College of Obstetricians and Gynecologists: Washington, DC.

25. Mecca L. 2003. Personal communication.

26. Walker R, Turnbull D, Wilkinson C. 2002. Strategies to address global cesarean section rates: a review of the evidence. *Birth*, 29(1):28–39.

27. Nolson FC. 1990. International differences in the use of obstectric interventions. *JAMA*, 263(24):3286–3291.

28. Frith M. 2003. MP's to quiz mothers on rise in caesareans. *Evening Standard*. London. Jan 16, 2003 (via Internet).

29. Belizan JM, Althabe F, Barros FC, et al. 1999. Rates and implications of caesarean sections in Latin America: Ecological study. *BMJ* 319(7222):1397–1400.

30. Pugin E. 2002. *Rising CS Rates Globally and in Chile: Impact on Breastfeeding*. Presentation at: WABA Second Global Forum. Arusha, Tanzania, September 2002.

31. International Cesarean Awareness Network (ICAN), Inc. website. *www.ican.org*. International Cesarean and VBAC rates (updated March 2002).

32. Cai W-W, Marks JS, Chen C, et al. 1998. Increased cesarean section rates and emerging patterns of health insurance in Shanghai, China. *Am J Pubic Health*, 88:77–80.

33. Wagner M. 2000. Choosing cesarean section. *Lancet* 356:1677–1680.

34. Pettiti D, Cefano RC, Sapiro S, et al. 1982. In hospital maternal mortality in the United Sates: Time trend and relation to method of delivery. *Obstet Gynecol*, 59:6–11.

35. Mbabane Government Hospital/Swaziland Ministry of Health, Central Statistics Office. Causes of maternal deaths. 1988.

36. Procianoy RS, Fernandes-Fillro PH, Lazaro L, et al. 1984. Factors affecting breastfeeding: The influence of caesarean section. *J Trop Pediatr*, 30:39–42.
37. Samuels SE, Margen S, Schoen EJ. 1985. Incidence and duration of breastfeeding in a health maintenance organization population. *Am J Clin Nutr*, 42:504–510.
38. Vestermark V, Hogdell CK, Birch M, et al. 1990. Breastfeeding duration following cesarean and vaginal births. *J Nurse Midwif*, 33(4):159–164.
39. Janke JR. 1988. Breastfeeding duration following cesarean and vaginal births. *J Nurse Midwif*, 33(4):159–164.
40. Sozmen M. 1992. Effects of early suckling of cesarean-born babies on lactation. *Biol Neonate*, 62:67–68.
41. Otamiri G, Berg G, Leden T, et al. 1991. Delayed neurological adaptation in infants delivered by elective cesarean section and the relation to catecholamine levels. *Early Hum Dev*, 26:51–60.
42. Nissen E, Uvnas-Moberg K, Svensson K, et al. 1996. Different patterns of oxytocin prolactin but not cortisol release during breastfeeding in women delivered by cesarean section or by the vaginal route. *Early Hum Dev*, 45:103–118.
43. Rowe-Murray H, and Fisher J. 2001. Operative intervention in delivery is associated with compromised early mother-infant interaction. *Br J Obstet Gynecol*, 108:1068–1075.
44. Frieman J. 2000. Why I wanted a C-section. *Self*, 6:96–99.
45. Wagner M. 1994. *Pursuing the Birth Machine: The Search for Appropriate Birth Technology*. Sydney: ACE Graphics.
46. WHO. 1981. *International Code of Marketing Breast-milk Substitutes*. Geneva: WHO.

CHAPTER 9

FEAR AND STRESS IN CHILDBIRTH AND BREASTFEEDING

"Reduced neo-cortex activity—as if 'going to another planet'—is a most important aspect of birth physiology from a practical point of view."

Michel Odent, 1999

Background and Early Research

Chapter 2 highlighted the importance of oxytocin (from the Greek, meaning *rapid labor*) in childbirth and lactation and also outlined the antagonistic effect that stressful events can have on its action in mammals. The fact that disturbances, stress, and fear affect hormonal mechanisms governing the onset and progress of normal labor and subsequent mothering behavior were well recognized decades ago. These early studies were on mice, commonly used in the 1960s as a surrogate model for human labor mechanisms.[1] Newton established that environmental disturbances could profoundly affect the course of labor and early mothering in lab animals, and she hypothesized that these effects were also important in humans.

Newton and Newton were pioneers four decades ago in documenting that the childbirth environment mattered. They prospectively studied differing types of labor support and pain relief for mothers in labor and the impact of interaction immediately after delivery with their newborns.[2] The discomfort of labor was controlled by three methods: "kind solicitous treatment," "attention to physical comfort positions changes, etc.," and "lighter analgesics for pain." [Author's note: This "light" analgesic included 50 mg of Demerol; however, only 3% of subjects received this medication]. An observation form and methodology previously utilized by these researchers was used to rate mothers' reactions to their babies. Findings were that mothers who received solicitous care were most likely to show acceptance of their newborns. The keywords given by the authors in their summary of the responses from the mothers about supportive care were "kindness, cooperation, and calmness."

Research on Stress Hormones and Human Birth

A decade after these early studies, a nurse researcher, Regina Lederman, and her associates demonstrated the hormonal interconnection between stress hormones and labor. They prospectively sampled blood catecholamine levels from healthy primiparous laboring mothers and established that low levels of adrenaline in early labor foster faster, easier progress compared to high levels of adrenaline.[3] In a follow-on study they established a relationship between high adrenaline levels in labor and lower uterine contractibility and longer second stage.[4] In a further study, they looked at multiple variables and established that high blood adrenaline in mothers in labor (this time the sample was healthy multiparous women, rather than primiparous) was associated with increased stress as evaluated by an unbiased observer. In addition there was increased perceived stress by the mother herself, decrease in strength of labor contractions as measured by internal pressure catheters, and finally a "less reassuring" fetal monitoring tracing, suggesting a decrease in fetal well being.[5]

Stress, Pain, and Self-Esteem

Studies on human labor established that endogenous opioids called beta-endorphins are secreted during labor, increase with intensity of contractions, and reach peaks as delivery draws near.[6-8] Although beta-endorphins do not eliminate labor pain, their effects in most women are to "blunt" or modulate the pain.[9] Also established is the finding that maternal plasma beta-endorphin levels during labor fall dramatically when epidural anesthesia is administered.[10] When an epidural is placed in labor, it seems to turn off the natural pain modulation afforded by beta-endorphins (see Figure 9-1). The anesthesia provided by epidural, while often effective, also requires a number of other interventions (discussed at some length in other chapters) that may interfere with breastfeeding.

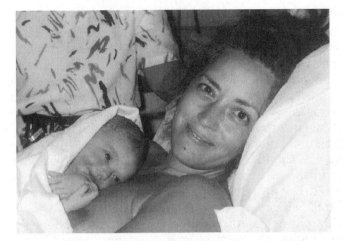

FIGURE 9-1   Lisa had a long labor with her first baby. She did not use any medication, took warm showers, walked, and used position changes. Her husband, a close friend, and a midwife supported her throughout labor. Here, minutes after birth in a hospital, she and her baby show evidence that they have circulating catecholamines and beta-endorphins: both have dilated pupils, an alert, calm demeanor, and mother seems to be in total bliss. The baby went to breast within 30 minutes. *Photo by Jere Graham, 1998.*

At about this same time, Klaus and Kennel's research on mother-infant bonding[11] reinforced the importance of a supportive environment before, during, and after delivery to foster bonding between the infant, the new mother, and sometimes the new father. Low anxiety would imply higher self-confidence, self-control, and self-esteem. The importance of this bonding period will be discussed in more depth in Chapter 10, but the discussion in Chapter 3 on support in labor documents that women who are supported in labor generally feel greater control and cope better with the pain and are better prepared for breastfeeding and mothering.

A prospective study in Utah looked at how women perceived their birth experiences after labor pain anesthesia with or without epidural.[12] The study used two socioeconomic ally homogeneous cohorts of healthy women at term, 45 of whom chose epidural anesthesia in labor and 44 who had no epidural (this group had either no medicines at all or local anesthetic for second stage). Actual labor interventions incurred by the two groups differed substantially, with the epidural versus nonepidural group having more oxytocin augmentation (46% versus 9%), electronic fetal monitoring (90% versus 66%), urinary catheterizations (58%

versus 7%), forceps deliveries (56% versus 5%), and episiotomies (85% versus 68%). All mothers were interviewed at 36 hours after delivery with a questionnaire based on previously tested psychological, personality, and pain perception scales. Findings were that mothers who had had epidurals had greater fear of the childbirth process, greater belief in powerful others, and were more passive. Only 2% of the epidural group mentioned safety of the baby as a primary motivation compared with 33% of the nonepidural labor management group. The fact that the epidural group was significantly younger (average age 20 years versus 26 years in the nonepidural group) may account for some of these findings. These findings support a profile of women who choose epidural, which includes fear of pain, need to give decision-making power to others, and lack of understanding that labor interventions may negatively impact the newborn. There is no information in this study about the infants' condition at birth or about feeding choice, so no additional conclusions can be drawn.

Lowe, an obstetrical nurse researcher, reviewed the literature on women's perception of pain in labor in relationship to their own self-confidence and ability to cope.[13] The author uses a "self-efficacy" model in which an individual evaluates her own capability to cope with stressful situations that develop during childbirth and to perform required behaviors. Research findings suggest that labor is perceived as less painful by a woman if she feels confident in her own coping mechanisms before and during labor. Findings reinforce the critical role that labor care attendants play in building (or undermining) a mother's self-confidence. The discussion also notes that the lack of a "significant other," some labor complications, and inconsistencies in information from care providers can undermine the self-efficacy of a laboring woman.

Data from the Mexico City study on labor support (see Chapter 3) allowed for a tandem qualitative study in which in-depth interviews were conducted early in the postpartum period with eight mothers from the "supported in labor" cohort and eight who received "routine care."[14] The most significant finding was that women who had a doula felt they had taken an active part in their labor, had more control, coped better with pain, and helped their own birth along. The authors conclude: "...the women in the group with a doula had a greater sense of participation and a higher self-esteem." Anxiety, loss of control, fear, and pain can all evoke a stress response that can adversely affect the progress of labor, often necessitating oxytocin or other interventions and affecting breastfeeding readiness.

Birth trauma is usually a term used to describe adverse newborn outcomes, but it can also be expanded to describe symptoms in the mother. A recent prospective longitudinal study in Australia by Creedy, et al, shows a strong relationship between childbirth events and acute maternal trauma symptoms.[15] A culturally diverse group of 499 pregnant women in their last trimester completed questionnaires in the antenatal clinic. Women were excluded if they had past history of trauma. Mothers were followed up with phone interviews at 4-6 weeks postpartum to explore their perceptions of the care they had received and presence of intrapartum traumatic events. One in three women (33%) identified a traumatic birthing event and exhibited three or more trauma symptoms. These symptoms were most commonly extreme pain, fear for her own or her baby's life, or both, and a perceived "lack of care." Almost 6% of the postpartum mothers interviewed met criteria for acute posttraumatic stress disorder. The level of obstetrical intervention was a strong predictor of acute trauma symptoms with emergency CS and forceps delivery being highly correlated. No information about mothering behavior or infant feeding patterns is reported in this study.

Another recent prospective longitudinal study in the United States looked at prevalence and predictors of psychological trauma in childbirth.[16] One hundred and three women were completed a survey in late pregnancy and were interviewed at 4 weeks postpartum. Findings were similar to the Creedy study in that 34% of women reported the childbirth experience as traumatic. Two women developed all the symptoms associated with posttraumatic stress disorder and almost one third of the women exhibited at least some symptoms of this disorder. Regression analysis to determine predictors of this trauma showed that in addition to preexisting factors, such as prior history of sexual abuse, labor factors included: pain in first stage of labor; feelings of powerlessness; medical interventions, including cesarean section; and interpersonal interactions with medical personnel.

Maternal Stress Hormones: Harmful or Helpful for Baby?

In the mid 1980s, Lagercrantz and Slotkin reviewed all the research, including their own, on stress hormones, and how they impact the mother, the fetus in labor, and the newborn in the early postpartum.[17] Careful analysis of 20 years of evidence at that point suggested a synergistic effect of maternal catecholamines, which increase in concentration as the labor strength increases,

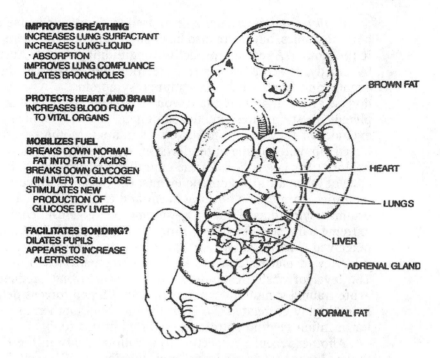

IMPROVES BREATHING
INCREASES LUNG SURFACTANT
INCREASES LUNG-LIQUID
  ABSORPTION
IMPROVES LUNG COMPLIANCE
DILATES BRONCHIOLES

PROTECTS HEART AND BRAIN
INCREASES BLOOD FLOW
  TO VITAL ORGANS

MOBILIZES FUEL
BREAKS DOWN NORMAL
  FAT INTO FATTY ACIDS
BREAKS DOWN GLYCOGEN
  (IN LIVER) TO GLUCOSE
STIMULATES NEW
  PRODUCTION OF
  GLUCOSE BY LIVER

FACILITATES BONDING?
DILATES PUPILS
APPEARS TO INCREASE
  ALERTNESS

BROWN FAT

HEART

LUNGS

LIVER

ADRENAL GLAND

NORMAL FAT

FIGURE 9-2 Adaptational effects of a catacholamine surge during delivery include promotion of normal breathing, alteration of blood flow to protect heart and brain against potential asphyxia, immediate mobilization of fuel for energy, and possibly enhancement of maternal-infant attachment. In general, the effects prepare the body to maintain homeostasis (stable functioning) at birth even if the neonate is exposed to such adversity as oxygen deprivation. *Adapted from: Lagercrantz and Slotkin, 1986.*[17] © Patricia J. Wynne.

cross the placental barrier to the fetal circulation, and allow for optimal preparation for life outside the womb (see Figure 9-2). This hormonal surge in the mother and then her unborn baby, allows for clearing the newborn's lungs, promotion of normal extrauterine breathing, mobilization of brown fat to be available for warmth and calories, provision of a rich supply of blood to the newborn's heart and brain, and may promote attachment behavior between mother and her newborn. These authors note that infants born by cesarean section are known to have breathing difficulties due to both inadequate absorption of lung liquid at birth and inadequate production of surfactant, the "soapy" substance that enables the collapsed lung in the fetal state to expand during the newborn's first breath.

Italian researchers have produced additional evidence that a natural "purpose" exists for the pain of labor and childbirth. The stress and coping hormones secreted as a result cross over to the fetus and newborn. Zanardo and associates noted that beta-endorphins are much higher in the first and second stages of labor compared to pregnancy.[18] They looked at beta-endorphin concentrations in the colostrum of two study groups: 14 healthy mothers at term who delivered naturally (vaginally without medication) and 14 who delivered by elective cesarean section under epidural anesthesia. In all mothers, colostral milk was extracted and analyzed for presence of beta-endorphins on day 4 postpartum. Findings were that colostral beta-endorphins were significantly higher in the vaginally delivered mothers compared to those delivered by planned cesarean section.

In a subsequent study, the same researchers sampled beta-endorphins in colostrum and transitional breast milk at 4, 10, and 30 days postpartum of three groups of mothers: one group vaginally delivered at term, one group vaginally delivered preterm (35.6 weeks +/− 0.3 days), and a third group delivered at term by elective cesarean section.[19] Findings, similar to their earlier study, were that beta-endorphins are significantly higher in colostrums of vaginally delivered mothers, with the preterm deliveries showing colostrums with the highest concentrations. In this group the higher concentrations lasted to day 10 postpartum. At 30 days postpartum there was no differences among the groups (see Figure 9-3) These authors hypothesize that elevated beta-endorphin levels in colostrum and transitional milk may be involved with postpartum adaptation to stress and possible other conditions. The finding that levels are even higher and sustained longer in mothers of preterm infants, who would have greater adaptations to make, suggests a special adaptation to the needs of the preterm infant. The authors also hypothesize that neonates delivered after long labor, either vaginally or by cesarean section, may be at a disadvantage in beta-endorphin availability for their babies. This can occur if there is delay in milk secretion or difficulty in expressing colostrum and transitional breast milk.

Labor Stress and Lactogenesis

Recent studies have investigated the hypothesis that stress in labor may affect breastfeeding. In a peri-urban population in northern California, Chen studied the relationship between birth

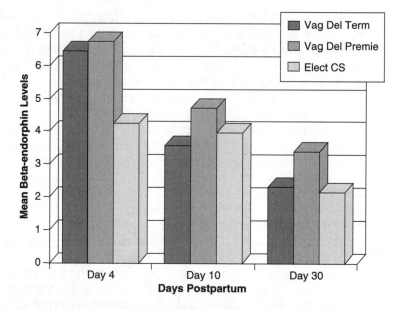

FIGURE 9-3 Mean beta-endorphin levels in colostrum and transitional milk, by type of delivery. *Adapted from Zanardo et al., 2001b.*[18]

and lactation in 40 healthy pregnant women at term, with a particular emphasis on events during labor and delivery, stress hormones, and lactation outcomes.[20] The power of this prospective study rests in the fact that key aspects of labor and delivery were directly observed, and stress hormones were measured during pregnancy, labor, delivery (maternal and cord blood), and during lactation, with several markers of lactogenesis tracked. Four outcomes were used as markers of onset of lactogenesis: the time when the subject first feels breast fullness, 24-hour milk volume on day 5 postpartum, milk lactose concentration on day 5 postpartum, and the appearance of casein in the milk. Findings were that at the time of delivery, women who had longer labors had greater levels of stress hormones in their blood as well as in the cord blood. In addition, a longer duration of labor was associated with maternal exhaustion and lower breastfeeding frequency on day 1. A longer duration of second stage of labor (not first stage) was associated with longer intervals between delivery and the first breastfeed. Primagravidas were also more likely to have longer labors, breastfed less often on the first day after delivery, felt breast fullness later, and had lower milk volume on day 5 postpartum. A schematic representation of this interrelationship is seen in Figure 9-4. A major flaw in this study is that researchers

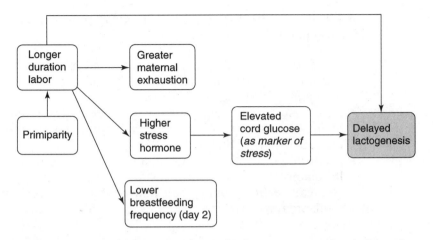

FIGURE 9-4   Possible causal pathways for factors associated with delayed lactogenesis. Based on timing of breast fullness, milk volume on day 5, and day of casein appearance. Women who had cesarean sections were excluded. Arrows denote significant interactions (p < 0.05) *Adapted with permission by the* American Journal of Clinical Nutrition © *Am J Clin Nutr. American Society for Clinical Nutrition.*

did not examine the role of the baby in effective milk removal as a possible confounding factor.

In a follow-on study, Dewey published data on factors related to delayed lactogenesis from a larger community-based sample of 280 mother-infant pairs who were recruited immediately after delivery.[21] Mothers were of mixed parity and all mothers in the study had healthy, single, term infants and were planning to breastfeed. Three outcome variables were used: infant sucking ability on day 1 and 3 as measured by the IBFAT score, infant weight change at day 3, and the timing of onset of lactation by the mother's perceived change in breast fullness. Trained professionals gave all mothers lactation guidance on days 3, 7, 14, and additional days as needed in the hospital and at home. Findings, after multivariate analysis, showed that with a high degree of consistency among the three markers for lactogenesis, both long duration of labor (both stage one and stage two) and urgent cesarean section were strongly related to delay in lactogenesis.

In the discussion of this research, Dewey notes that in both prolonged labor and urgent cesarean section, maternal stressors include physical stressors such as exhaustion and/or pain and emotional stressors such as anxiety. These maternal, infant, or combined stressors may contribute to delay in lactogenesis. Possible mechanisms proposed are:

- The direct relationship between stress and inhibition of oxytocin, if recurrent, could reduce milk production by reducing the emptying of the breast.
- Milk removal may not trigger lactogenesis stage II, but frequent interference with milk ejection could down-regulate the rate of milk synthesis.
- Labor and birth, if prolonged and/or if involved with stressful maternal or fetal conditions, including emergency cesarean section, could result in a newborn too weak, tired, or disorganized to latch on and suckle effectively.

Developing Countries and Resource-Poor Settings

Is stress in labor a hospital-based or "Western" phenomenon and do home births or community-based births automatically support a woman's emotional and psychological needs? As early as 1967, the anthropologist Margaret Mead, joined by Niles Newton, published some important observations on laboring patterns of two cultures in Central and South America. In one culture, the Cuña Indians of Central America, coitus and birth were viewed with shame, and labor and delivery was orchestrated by a medicine man who, though not present at the event, made medicinal teas which he gave to the midwives to administer. Labors were reported to be prolonged and agonizing. In contrast, these authors observed that the Siriono Indians in South America, among whom childbirth is considered to be a natural process, labored in their hammocks in communal huts. Family and friends attended a woman in labor and on average, her labor and delivery lasted one to three hours.[22]

Chapter 1 described the global strategies for a "safe motherhood" initiative aimed at reducing maternal mortality and morbidity, and explained that these strategies must also help the mother "feel safe." Global programs still largely fail to build in the "mother-friendly" pillar in the structure of safe motherhood for all. Other chapters have reviewed ways that developing countries and maternity settings with few resources could adapt the birth environment to reduce stress for the mother in labor.

It is helpful to look at one populous country that has tried to address both safe motherhood and mothers "feeling safe." Indonesia, with a population of over 230 million people, has a persist-ently high maternal mortality rate with 390/100,000 being the most quoted figure.[23] The government has recognized that the vast majority of rural Indonesians prefer delivery at home with a local traditional midwife or *dukun*. Between 1993 and 1999 there was a focused effort to train and dispatch over 55,000 nurse-mid-wives to rural villages all over Indonesia with the expectation that they would partner with or take over the work of the *dukun*. Often the newly posted midwife was very young, unmarried, childless, and clinically inexperienced and she had to work diligently to establish credibility and trust with the village to which she was assigned. Community acceptance of this young government mid-wife was only one of the challenges. Maternal-perinatal death audits in the large province of Central Java revealed that the gov-ernment referral hospitals were often poorly equipped, charged illegal fees in advance of care, and had staff who treated the women referred in labor very poorly.[24] The reputation of this poor care and commonplace mistreatment of patients led to very late referrals and frequent refusal of referral by the woman's family, even when there was a life-threatening condition. Many women (or the decision maker in their families) preferred to die at home in dignity rather than face the stress, fear, and insensitive care at a strange district hospital.[25]

To address this "mother unfriendly" situation in referral facil-ities, in 1995 health planners in Central Java began expansion of their existing Baby Friendly Hospital Initiative to include mother-friendly practices. "Mother Friendly Hospital" criteria were drafted that not only strengthened emergency obstetrical serv-ices, but also humanized birthing practices and addressed the need for culturally appropriate and supportive care in referral hospitals. For many hospitals this meant changing strict policies. Gradually, close family members were allowed into the labor room to encourage the mother in her local dialect, provide mas-sage, and overall to reduce stress in labor. In other instances this "friendliness" amounted to provision of clay pots so that the pla-centa, a culturally significant product of the birth to the Javanese, could be safely carried home for ritual burial (see Fig-ures 9-5 and 9-6). Follow-up investigation in 1997 showed that in district hospitals where the mother friendly hospital initiative was implemented, high-risk mothers were being brought in a timely manner, were being attended to immediately, were per-mitted to have a close relative in the maternity ward, were allowed to walk, and were provided with fluids in labor. The rou-tine episiotomy rate in one hospital dropped dramatically as a

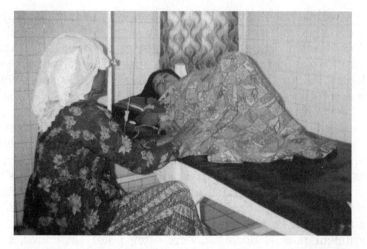

FIGURE 9-5 In Central Java, some district hospitals changed their routines to help combat high maternal mortality. This young mother was carrying a breech baby and agreed to come to the hospital because her mother was allowed to be with her. *Photo by Mary Kroeger, 1997.*

result of this initiative. The Baby Friendly Hospital practices continued, and in general, care for all mothers and newborns improved.[26]

Culture Lag, Research Gap, or Simply Ignoring the Evidence?

In 1988 in *Laboring Undisturbed*, Newton notes the continued lack of emphasis on research on the birthing "environment":

> In the 20 years since I have asked the question, the effect of environment on labor still tends to garner less research attention than do biochemical and surgical interventions. Two noteworthy programs, both open to high-risk and low-risk expectant women, have paid attention to developing a favorable environment for labor and delivery and reporting the results.[27]

The article cites as an exemplary model, the maternity center in Pithiviers, France (directed at that time by Michel Odent), where all mothers were accepted whether with or without risk factors, and there was a 6.6% cesarean section rate, a 5.2% vacuum rate, and a 6% episiotomy rate. Furthermore, less then 2% of the newborns needed to be removed from their mothers for special care.

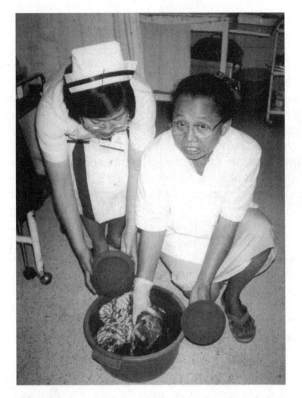

FIGURE 9-6   Other hospitals provide covered clay pots, which are given to the family with the placenta so that the proper ritual and burial at home can occur. Now more mothers agree to referral because they are receiving sensitive hospital care. *Photo by Mary Kroeger, 1997.*

Another noteworthy model cited at the time of this article was the midwifery service in North Central Bronx Hospital in New York City. This large inner-city hospital service, serving a lower socioeconomic, multiethnic, and immigrant population, including at risk-patients, still was able to protect the birth environment. Of the over 2600 deliveries in 1979, including low- and high-risk mothers, 88% of the births were normal, spontaneous vaginal deliveries.[28] The cesarean section rate was 9% and the instrumental delivery rate 2.3%; there were no elective inductions of labor and only 3% required oxytocin augmentation; 70% of all births were completely unmedicated; 74% delivered without an episiotomy, and 45% of these mothers delivered over completely intact perineum; 85% of the mothers gave birth in their labor beds and in an upright position, rather than on traditional delivery tables.

These impressive statistics, not found today in inner-city hospitals, were achieved by a policy of *protecting the birth environment* through low intervention, minimal use of labor medications, and mother-friendly care. Laboring mothers were accompanied by one to two companions of their choosing and they walked, ate, and drank in labor. Vaginal examinations were minimal and artificial rupture of membranes was rare. Newborn outcomes were equally impressive, with a neonatal mortality rate of 4.2/1000 for all infants over 1000 grams. No information on breastfeeding and infant feeding rates or outcomes are reported in the article; however, unpublished data from this study in 1979 show that 70–80% of the mothers were breastfeeding at the time of discharge.[29]

Childbirth free from unnecessary medical intervention and stress sets the stage for optimal breastfeeding. Newton's quotation at the beginning of this section reflected back two decades from 1988, to a skewed research emphasis on "biochemical and surgical interventions" rather than preserving normalcy in birth. Two decades after the Newton article, Michel Odent (as discussed in Chapter 2) continues to reflect on the seemingly intentional research gap in the study of normal childbirth.[30] Why are we stressing our mothers and newborns and undermining breastfeeding?

Summary Points for Protecting the Mother-Baby Continuum

- Studies in mammals, including humans, show that high levels of stress hormones interfere with oxytocin, interfere with normal labor progress, and are linked to adverse birth outcomes.
- Mothers want security and safety in labor and birth.
- Obstetrical interventions are correlated with perceived traumatic birth events.
- Newborns from vaginal delivery, with high levels of catecholamines from the maternal circulation, are better equipped to adapt to extrauterine life than those delivered by cesarean section.
- Growing evidence shows that stressful labor events are associated with less frequent suckling and later onset of lactogenesis, especially in first-time mothers.
- Evidence shows that endogenous opioids, beta-endorphins, are secreted in high concentrations during labor, peak close to delivery, and play a role in blunting the perceived pain of childbirth. Labor medications, including epidural anesthesia, block the normal secretion of maternal beta-endorphins during labor.

- Beta-endorphins are found in high concentrations in colostrum in vaginal delivery and may play a role in newborn adaptation to extrauterine stress.

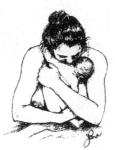

References

1. Newton N, Foshee D, Newton M. 1966. Parturient mice: Effects of environment on labor. *Science* 151:1560–1561.
2. Newton N, Newton M. 1962. Mother's reactions to their newborn babies. *JAMA* 181:206–210.
3. Lederman R, McCann D, Work B, et al. 1977. Endogenous plasma epinephrine and norepinephrine in last trimester and labor. *Am J Obstet. Gynecol* 129:5–8.
4. Lederman R, Lederman E, Work B, et al. 1978. The relationship of maternal anxiety, plasma catecholamines and plasma cortisol to progress in labor. *Am J Obstet Gynecol* 78:495–499.
5. Lederman R, Lederman E, Work B. 1985. Anxiety and epinephrine in multiparous women in labor: Relationship to duration of labor and fetal heart rate patterns. *Am J Obstet Gynecol* 153:870–877.
6. Facchinetti F, Centini G, Parrini D, et al. 1982. Opioid plasma levels during labor. *Gynecol Obstet Invest* 13(3):155–163.
7. Thomas TA, Fletcher JE, Hill RG. 1982. Influence of medication, pain, and progress in labor on plasma endorphin-like immunoreactivity. *Br J Anaesth* 54(4):401–408.
8. Gintzler A. 1980. Endorphin-mediated increases in pain threshold during pregnancy. *Science* 210:193–195.
9. Cahill CA. 1989. Beta-endorphin levels during pregnancy and labor: A role in pain modulation? *Nurs Res* 38(4):200–203.
10. Hoffman DI, Abboud TK, Haase HR, et al. 1984. Plasma beta-endorphin concentrations prior to and during pregnancy, in labor and after delivery. *Am J Obstet Gynecol* 150(5, part I):492–496.

11. Klaus M, Kennell J, 1983. *Bonding the Beginning of Parent-Infant Attachment.* St. Louis: C.V. Mosby.

12. Poore M, and Foster JC. 1985. Epidural and no epidural anesthesia: Differences between mothers and their experience of birth. *Birth* 12(4):205–212.

13. Lowe N. 1991. Maternal confidence coping with labor: A self-efficacy concept. *JOGNN* 20(6):457–463.

14. Campero L, Garcia C, Diaz C, et al. 1998. "Alone I wouldn't have known what to do": A qualitative study on social support during labor and delivery in Mexico. *Soc Sci Medicine* 47(3):395–403.

15. Creedy D, Shochet IM, Horsfall J. 2000. Childbirth and the development of acute trauma symptoms: Incidence and contributing factors. *Birth* 27(2):104–111.

16. Soet J, Brack, G, Dilorio C. 2003. Prevalence and Predictors of Women's Experience of Psychological Trauma During Childbirth. *Birth* 30(1):36–46.

17. Lagercrantz H, Slotkin TA. 1986. The stress of being born. *Scientific American* 254:91–102.

18. Zanardo V, Nicolussi S, Giacomin C, et al. 2001a. Labor pain effects on colostral milk beta-endorphins concentrations of lactating mothers. *Biol Neonate* 79(2):87–90.

19. Zanardo V, Nicolussi S, Carlo G, et al. 2001b. Beta-endorphin concentrations in human milk. *J Pediatr Gastroenterol Nutr* 33(2):160–164.

20. Chen DC, Nommsen-Rivers L, Dewey K, et al. 1998. Stress during labor and delivery and early lactation performance. *Am J Clin Nutr* 68:335–344.

21. Dewey KG. 2001. Maternal and fetal stress are associated with impaired lactogenesis. *J. Nutri.* 131:3012S–3015S.

22. Mead M, Newton N. 1967. Cultural patterning in perinatal behavior. In: Richardson SA and Guttmacher AF (eds.) *Childbearing: Its Social and Psychological Aspects.* Baltimore: Williams and Wilkins, 142–144.

23. Daly P. 2000. *Reproductive Health in Indonesia: The Challenges and Risks Ahead.* Draft Report to the World Bank. Washington, DC.

24. Kroeger M. 1996. *Final Report on Technical Assistance to the CHN III Project.* Semarang: Central Java, Department of Health, Central Java, Indonesia.

25. Iskander MB, et al. 1996. *Unraveling the Mysteries of Maternal Death in West Java: Reexamining the Witnesses.* Depok: Center for Health Research, Research Institute, University of Indonesia.

26. Miller S, and Kroeger M. 1997. *Trip Report on Consultancy to Indonesia,* July 1997. Chapel Hill, North Carolina: PRIME/INTRAH.
27. Newton N. 1988. Laboring Undisturbed. *Psychology Today* 15:35–38.
28. Haire DB. 1981. Improving outcome of pregnancy through increased utilization of midwives. *J Nurse-Midwifery* 26(1):5–8.
29. Haire DB. 2003. Personal communication.
30. Odent M. 2000. Between circular and cul-de-sac epidemiology. *Lancet* 355(9212):1371.

CHAPTER 10

IMMEDIATE SKIN-TO-SKIN CONTACT AFTER BIRTH

"A hot sweet smell fills the hut, and during the next two contractions the young woman barely works at all, letting her body slowly squeeze the infant out, one slippery shoulder at a time.... It sputters, cries once, and begins to breathe on its own, its body still half immersed in the mother."

Suzanne Arms, 1975

Evidence Is Established

Immediate mother-baby contact after birth has been firmly established as evidence-based practice that supports breastfeeding. The Baby Friendly Hospital Initiative (BFHI), implemented on a global scale since 1992, introduced this practice in maternity facilities as the recommended standard of immediate post delivery care. Step Four of the Ten Steps to Successful Breastfeeding states, "Help mothers initiate breast-feeding within half-hour of birth."[1] Additional scientific documentation has reinforced this recommendation in the *Evidence for the Ten Steps*, which reviewed the older evidence and cited additional studies.[2]

The normal newborn has a "recovery period" right after birth of about 5–30 minutes. Then the baby, if undisturbed and left on the mother's abdomen, begins to look for and crawl up to the mother's nipple.[3] Newer research, which continues to underscore the critical nature of this period, describes specific coordinated patterns of newborn hand and sucking movements and massage of the mother's breasts in unmedicated undisturbed infants.[4,5] During this time the infant's stress hormone levels (catecholamines) are high,[6] pupils are dilated, reflexes are keen, and the newborn is in a wide-awake, alert state. Newer studies show that there are additional adaptive prebreastfeeding behaviors in the first hour after delivery when an infant is left undisturbed on the mother's abdomen. These include fist clenching, hand-to-mouth movements, rooting, sucking, and actual latch-on.[7] The newborn olfactory responses are cued into the smell of amniotic fluid and the smell of the mother's breasts before washing.[8,9] This heightened sense of smell may lead the newborn to crawl to the mother's breast and find the nipple.

There is a similar "sensitive period" for the mother, during which she too is "looking" for her newborn and is receptive to the first feed. Newton has described this mothering behavior and the role of oxytocin as a hormone of nurturing and love.[10] The studies on continuous support in labor suggest that a mother who has felt emotional support is better able to receive and care for her baby.[11] Klaus and Kennell have written extensively on the critical first few hours or "bonding period" for the newborn, and have also pioneered in the promotion of doula support in labor. In their popular book written for consumers, *Mothering the Mother,* Klaus, Kennell, and Klaus note:

> There is a remarkable similarity between the results of the doula support in the South African study [Hofmeyr, 1991][11] and the behavior of mothers given early and increased contact with their infants (the so-called bonding studies). Both groups of mothers showed or reported increased affection and attention to their babies, had increased desire to stay home and care for their infants in the first weeks, and were more likely to pick up their babies whenever they were crying. These mothers also tended to breastfeed more often and longer. Such striking differences at six weeks later from such a short period of support is a reminder that the period of labor is a time when the mother is especially sensitive to environmental factors and open to learning and growth. [12]

This chapter builds on the evidence presented at greater length in preceding chapters, and reviews newer findings that continue to strengthen the case for early and sustained mother-baby contact. Also discussed are the difficulties that are implicitly built into the modern birth environment, both in the Western setting with rising medical interventions and cesaraen section rates, and in the developing world, where cultural practices are hard to change.

Colostrum and Civilization

From ancient times there has been interference with the first moments after birth and immediate removal of the baby from the mother. Odent speculates in his paper, "Colostrum and Civilization," that disturbance in the early moments after birth may be historically linked to the evolution of humankind as a warrior species, who drive to carve territory and eliminate foreign tribes.[13] He writes:

> The most efficient way to make man a super-predator is to disturb the mother-newborn relationship. For a culture to claim colostrum is bad is an easy way of weakening this relationship and so, to do so, has, up to now, been an advantage in terms of selection. In fact the deprivation of colostrum is just one example of the cultural man's potential for cruelty towards the newborn baby, and for meddling in this relationship with his mother.

Odent describes the historical tendency of most cultures, both ancient and contemporary, to foster negative impressions of colostrum, terming it bad, dirty, pus-like, or poison. He also describes the few cultures where colostrum is not withheld and points out that these cultures are usually isolated from developed countries and have "a deeply rooted sense of ecology." Kitzinger has written about negative impressions of colostrum wherein it is seen in many cultures as "too strong or dangerous" and the newborn must be starved, fed other foods, or wet-nursed by another, usually a relative.[14]

The discarding of colostrum may have been a deliberate attempt to establish family lines. The author, who has worked widely with traditional midwives in developing countries, has found the influence of the traditional midwife to be significant in directing early breastfeeding practice. For example, in southern Malawi, one busy traditional midwife explained that she does not encourage colostrum right away. She waits to let the grandmother give the first feedings of thin corn porridge as the "greeting food" and also to establish the baby's place in the family line of inheritance (Figure 10-1). She explained that until recently she had discarded colostrum as "dirty," but recent training has changed her practice to encouraging colostrum. However, the corn porridge is still always given first.

A nonliterate traditional midwife cannot be criticized for her non-evidence-based practices. Unless she has received training, she may not understand the implications of withholding colostrum and of introducing an osmolarity-imbalanced, possibly contaminated, sugary corn gruel as a newborn's first feeds. It is not as easy to be forgiving of trained health workers, when the importance of early contact and colostrum has been well documented for several decades. In a dynamic medical seminar by Dr.

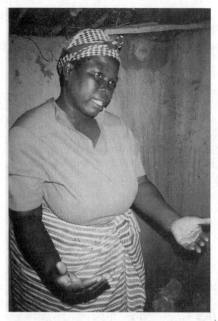

FIGURE 10-1 A busy homebirth midwife in Malawi describes her practice of withholding colostrum from the newborn and allowing the relatives to offer thin corn porridge as the first feed to greet the baby and establish inheritance lines. *Photo by Mary Kroeger, 2001.*

Muriel Sugarman, she articulated the urgent need for doctors to support early mother-baby contact.[15] She outlined the known benefits at the time:

- Implantation of mother's skin bacteria on the infant's skin. These homegrown bacteria are tolerated best by the newborn.
- Transfer of immunologic factors—both cellular and noncellular—via colostrum to the neonate's gastro-intestinal tract to prevent serious infections
- Completion of the spontaneous species-specific maternal behaviors described in human mothers by Klaus in 1970 and 1975
- Coordination of sucking at a period of heightened alertness to produce earlier milk production and more efficient early sucking by the infant
- Gut closure or sealing of the intestinal lining by colostrum to prevent or lessen passage of harmful bacteria or foreign protein molecules

- Production of endogenous oxytocin, which aids contraction of the uterus and expulsion of the placenta to minimize blood flow

A quarter of a century after this seminar, even more is known about the remarkable properties of colostrum. Yet this call to health care workers to ensure that maternity practices do not interfere with early breastfeeding is frequently not heeded, as routine medical procedures and nursing priorities come first. Given the importance of colostrum for the species-specific metabolic, immunologic, and nutritional role it plays in the human newborn, it is essential that every mother and father know what they are withholding of they "choose" not to breastfeed at least for a short time.

Timing of First Contact

The Global Baby Friendly Hospital Initiative assessment criteria for this Step Four state that:

> ...80% of mothers in the maternity ward who have had normal vaginal deliveries should confirm that within half-hour of birth they were given their babies to hold with skin contact, for at least 30 minutes, and offered help by a staff member to initiate breastfeeding. At least 50% of mothers who have had caesarean deliveries should confirm that within a half hour of being able to respond, they were given their babies to hold with skin contact.[16]

Recent updates by the UNICEF country offices sent to UNICEF Headquarters show that there are now more than 18,000 designated BFHI hospitals worldwide.[17] This should mean that babies are being put in their mother's arms and are initiating breastfeeding soon after birth all over the world. Yet reports of barriers and difficulties in implementing Step Four have been documented since the early years of implementation. Among the common barriers voiced were (and still are) lack of staff time in general, need to finish newborn procedures, the mother may drop the baby, need for episiotomy repair, the mother must be cleaned up first, need to move the mother from the delivery room, or the delivery room is too cold, to name a few.[18-20]

The United States adaptation of the global BFHI is implemented by a nonprofit agency called Baby-Friendly USA™. In

1993, a BFHI Feasibility Study was launched under the auspices of the Healthy Mothers, Healthy Babies Coalition, with funding from the Department of Health and Human Services. An Expert Work Group (EWG) was convened that met three times during 1993–1994 to discuss the feasibility of implementing BFHI in the United States. This EWG had representation from many sectors with conflicting interests and there was never full consensus about recommendations for criteria and assessment. A "minority report" of the EWG pointed out that the deliberations had not allowed for full discussion of issues.[21] As a result, Wellstart International, which had been very involved in the development of the global BFHI criteria and designation process, was asked to develop a BFHI process for the United States that could be pilot-tested in the initial round of assessments.[22]

For the most part, the U.S. initiative keeps the rigor of the global BFHI initiative. However, the wording of Step Four was changed to read: "Help all mothers initiate breast-feeding within one hour of birth." The rationale for this change was based on selected studies which suggested a broader range in timing for first feed. One study from Sweden, of 72 mother-baby pairs, showed a mean latch-on time of 49 minutes.[23] Another Swedish study also confirmed first suckling within an hour.[24] Accepting this "shift" in the timing of a physiologic mean of readiness for first suckling did not take into consideration the fact that more than half of the mothers in one study, and nearly half in the other, had received narcotics in labor. Other research was not solicited, it seems, because a randomized controlled trial in Malawi published in *Lancet* at the same time (1989) showed the average timing for 76 unmediated infants in a large general hospital city was an average of 7.25 minutes, with all babies latching on by 20 minutes after birth.[25]

In 1999, the International Lactation Consultant Association (ILCA) published its pamphlet, *Evidenced-Based Guidelines for Breastfeeding Management during the First Fourteen Days,* which includes reviews of additional evidence-based studies, although no new studies were included for Step Four. The wording of the ILCA "Management Strategy" for this step is: "facilitating breastfeeding as soon as possible after birth, ideally within the first 2 hours."[26]

Both the U.S. wording for the Ten Steps and the more recent ILCA recommendation have not used additional research other than the Swedish studies for shifting the period beyond 30 minutes. The global BFHI program also reevaluated the wording of this step, but decided it was best to leave the global Ten Steps as they are.[27] A guidance document to UNICEF field offices on reassessing BFHI states:

> If [baby and mother] are in continuous, undisturbed skin-to-skin contact from a few minutes after birth, the infant takes the breast at his or her own speed. The average time for an infant to attach spontaneously to the breast and suckle is about 55 minutes after birth, and in most cases it will happen within two hours. Evidence-based new practices do not hurry the newborn to the breast, they give healthy newborns uninterrupted full skin-to-skin contact with the mother in peaceful, warm conditions, allowing the baby to remain unwrapped and to move freely toward the breast.[28]

Is timing a small detail? This first 60 minutes are critical, and a vast body of science on imprinting in other mammals suggests that timing can determine the whole future of mothering. The "sensitive period" in humans seems to be relatively short, and standard lactation texts talk of the "deep sleep" that a baby lapses into after birth. Much interruption of mother and baby in that normal transition period can occur in 30 or 60 minutes. The Righard study showed that even weighing is not a benign interruption (Figure 10-2).

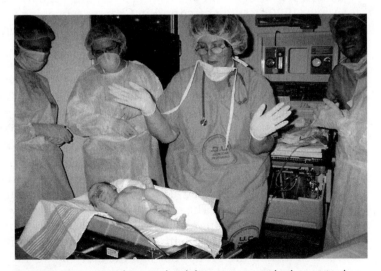

FIGURE 10-2 Weighing in the delivery room and other procedures are still common in U.S. hospitals. Numerous others may handle the newborn before she reaches her mother's arms. *Photo by Mary Kroeger, San Francisco 1998.*

Skin-to-Skin Contact: Selected Remarkable Findings

There is considerable literature from international studies, large and small, that documents evidence for early, uninterrupted, skin-to-skin contact of mother and baby. A few of them are highlighted in the following paragraphs.

- *Skin-to-skin contact prolongs breastfeeding and improves mothering (1977):* A classic study in Sweden in 1977 pointed the way to changing standard hospital routines, which at that time required separation of mother and baby at birth, four hourly feedings on schedule, test weighing of babies to make sure they had enough breast milk, and supplementation if they were considered underfed.[29] Two groups of mother-baby pairs, 21 in the early contact group and 20 in the routine care group, were followed in the hospital and up to three months afterwards. The test group had skin-to-skin contact and early suckling within the first hour of birth. Findings were that the median duration of breastfeeding was increased by 2 ½ months in the early contact group and that the "co-operative" relationship between mother and baby was improved. At 3 months postpartum, mothers were more likely to feed the baby at night than control mothers and deemed night feed "less of a problem."

- *Inborn self-attachment behavior (1990):* The Righard and Alade (1990)[30] study discussed in Chapter 6 remains one of the most important studies to date because of the inborn behaviors described when mothers and newborns have uninterrupted contact. Significant findings are that even "simple" procedures such as weighing and bathing create detrimental impact on first suckling. Discussed more thoroughly in Chapter 6 is the additional significant finding that narcotic analgesia also negatively impacts this inborn feeding behavior.

- *Short contact with nipple makes a difference (1990):* A study in Sweden tested effects of early nipple contact and suckling with two groups of healthy mother-baby pairs.[31] In the control group were 32 pairs with early contact skin-to-skin but no suckling. The study group were 25 pairs with the same arrangement, but also with contact between baby's lips and mother's nipple and with suckling encouraged. Findings showed that in the group that had the early lip-to-nipple contact, mothers left their babies in the nursery an average of 100 minutes a day less than the control mothers. Also, the study mothers showed higher maternal plasma gastrin levels, suggesting neuroendocrine functions were influenced by this early nipple contact.

- *Suckling influences gastrointestinal hormones (1989–1998):* When an infant suckles there is an outpouring of 19 gastrointestinal hormones, including gastrin, insulin, and cholecystokinin.[32] These hormones are known to stimulate newborn gut villi growth and enhance capacity for absorbing nutrients. Cholecystokinin (CCK), produced in both mother and baby during breastfeeding, is a gastrointestinal hormone that enhances digestion and also is associated with the "sleepy, full feeling."[33–35] When a baby stops suckling and comes spontaneously off the breast, CCK levels are high. Ten minutes later they have dropped. At two days of age CCK is high, perhaps as an adaptive mechanism for ensuring the infant is not distressed by hunger as the colostrum is transitioning to mature milk.

- *Preference for unwashed breast (1994, 2001):* Varendi and associates have studied the tendency for newborn mammals to be attracted to the smell of amniotic fluid and have tested this finding in human infants. In one study, 30 mother-baby pairs were kept together after delivery. Mothers had one breast washed and left the other unwashed. Temperatures of both breasts were the same. In moving towards the breast to prepare to suckle, 22 of the 30 infants preferred the unwashed breast.[36] In another study, 22 babies were placed in a cot with a breast pad, which carried the mother's odor, placed 17 inches from the baby's nose. The same infants, in a second trial, were placed 17 inches from a clean pad that had not come in contact with the mother. More babies moved towards the breast odor pad than the clean pad.[37] These authors conclude that the newborn has highly developed olfactory senses and preferentially responds to the odors of amniotic fluid and the mother's breast, as opposed to washed or clean items.

- *Kangaroo mother care (KMC) for premature infants (1983–2002):* The model of KMC was first developed and described in Bogotá, Colombia by Rey and Martinez (1983).[38] This method stabilizes premature infants through early and prolonged skin-to-skin contact in a kangaroo position between the mother's breasts. Ideally, exclusive breastfeeding is the feeding method. The KMC method was initially promoted as cost-effective for settings and countries that do not have the resources for incubators and warming cots, but over 20 years of research have proved it equally effective in developed country settings. KMC, with continuous skin-to skin contact between a premature baby and its kangaroo "mother," has been found to stabilize and regularize heart rate[39] and respiratory rate,[40] and regulates temperature faster than a radiant warmer.[41] KMC results in less crying[42] and has been shown to induce deeper sleep, including sleep with the delta brush brainwave pattern that is associated with synapse formation.[43] KMC promotes self-regulation in premature infants, and at 3 and 6 months after delivery they have better emotional and cognitive regulatory abilities and more efficient arousal.[44] KMC babies are twice as likely to breastfeed compared with incubator babies (82% versus 45% in one study). KMC mothers produced 60% more milk than mothers of incubated babies. In another study, a strong linear relationship was shown in increased breast milk production compared with controls in mothers who had initiated holding skin-to-skin in the first month after birth.[45] Mothers practicing KMC sleep better and have a deeper sense of well-being in that they "are doing something" for their premature baby.[46]

- *Analgesia effect of breastfeeding in term neonates (2003):* In a randomized controlled trial, 180 term babies who were to undergo venepuncture were randomized to breastfeeding, or, while being held in the mother's arms, were given glucose feed plus pacifier, sterile water, or no feed. Blinded evaluators of videotapes of each baby analyzed the levels of pain response during the procedure. There was a high level of significance to the soothing effects of breastfeeding and glucose plus pacifier compared with holding alone or with water.[47]

Box 10-1   Biological Nurturing: A Model of Care That Supports the Physiology of Metabolic Transition

Suzanne Colson, a nurse-midwife-researcher, is part of a team of doctors investigating metabolic transition in the newborn. Any baby in the United Kingdom who is born preterm or small for gestational age is considered at risk of hypoglycemia and is monitored closely during the first days. This monitoring includes routine blood sugar testing and complementary formula feeds after breastfeeding.

Colson and colleagues have proposed a model of care to address physiologic hypoglycemia and other aspects of postnatal adaptation. Called "Biological Nurturing," the theoretical framework is similar to kangaroo mother care with one important difference: biological nurturing does not have to be carried out skin-to-skin. Mothers are offered the choice and many choose to be lightly dressed. The model involves the following approaches.

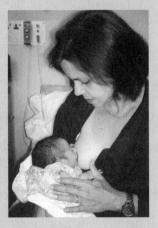

Figure 10-3   Having a mouthful of colostrum triggers a swallow, then a suck, and then the cycle repeats. Sleeping and latched onto the breast reinforces breastfeeding reflexes. *Photo by Suzanne Colson ©*

Biological Nurturing for the Baby

- Sleeping in arms, mouthing, licking, smelling, nuzzling, and nesting at the breast
- Groping and rooting at the breast
- Latching onto the breast
- Sucking, swallowing through active feeding

Biological Nurturing for the Mother

- Holding the baby so that face, chest, abdomen, and legs are closely flexed around a maternal body contour
- Offering unrestricted access to the breast with as much skin-to-skin contact as desired

Colson describes the metabolic transitioning of the newborn after birth as a shift from glucose to fat metabolism. She notes that fetal life is dominated by insulin, and it is used as a growth hormone *in utero* rather than as a metabolic regulator. When the baby is born, it comes into the world "well-fed." With the cutting of the cord, the constant supply of glucose stops, neonatal blood glucose levels drop, and the newborn's glycogen and fat stores are utilized in the first days to meet the needs of the newborn. In the first days, the baby learns how to breastfeed efficiently and stimulates the extrauterine

continued

Box 10-1 continued

food source: breast milk. The volume and content of early colostral milk meets the healthy newborn's requirements and larger volumes (as in formula feeds) may actually force the baby to "glug" and possibly overfill its small stomach, resulting in unnecessary vomiting.

Hypoglycemia in the newborn is overdiagnosed, according to Colson. She notes that bedside screening for hypoglycemia is unreliable and it is difficult to define hypoglycemia by using numbers, as the condition is a continuum that varies from baby to baby. During the first three postnatal days, the main threats to maintaining normal blood glucose levels are cold, stress, infant crying, and hospital routines that interrupt frequent ingestion of the small "drips and drops" of the mother's colostrum. Fears over hypoglycemia in newborns result in hospital practices that could actually be harmful. Several metabolic studies have demonstrated that when neonatal blood sugar concentrations are physiologically low, the breastfed baby counter regulates. That is, ketone bodies are formed from beta-oxidation of fats found in mother's milk and from adipose tissue. This is called *suckling ketosis*. Ketone bodies are an alternative energy source for the neonatal brain. Giving artificial formula feeds does not always raise neonatal blood sugar concentrations, but giving artificial formula suppresses ketogenesis in an inverse relationship to the amount given. Healthy breastfed babies rarely require supplementation from a metabolic perspective. Supplementation can cause needless anxiety, and research demonstrates that it can negatively affect early mother-infant adjustment as well as breastfeeding.

In a qualitative study, 12 mother-baby pairs were followed from birth to time of discharge.[48] Newborns were healthy but moderately preterm or small for gestational age. The preterm infants had a mean gestational age of 35.3 weeks and mean birth weight of 2644 g. They were managed with routine testing for hypoglycemia, and with Biological Nurturing as described above. In the first 24 hours, the mean time for breast contact was 7 hours and 40 minutes. None were hypothermic, and although skin-to-skin care was suggested, mothers and babies were not undressed. All were breastfeeding exclusively at hospital discharge. Biological Nurturing was found to facilitate breastfeeding. At six postnatal weeks all were still breastfeeding, eleven exclusively.

Routines Surrounding Childbirth That Hurt the Newborn

Suctioning

Suctioning the newborn's mouth and nose during or right after delivery remains a routine step in management of normal delivery worldwide. The WHO guide for midwives and doctors includes "suction the baby's mouth and nose" as a routine step in normal delivery.[49] *A Guide to Effective Care in Pregnancy and Childbirth* states that "the practice of routine suctioning to remove secretions from the newborn's mouth and nasal passages has not been assessed in any clinical trials, and its value is uncertain."[50] The ACOG/AAP Perinatal guidelines state, "The neonate's mouth may be suctioned gently to remove excess mucus or blood. Although clear mucus is suctioned from the mouth routinely in most centers, there is no evidence to support the value of this practice."[51] The ACOG/AAP guidelines go on to recommend that in the case of meconium-stained fluid, there should always be suctioning and if the infant is "depressed" there should be intubation followed by deep suctioning (Figure 10-4). The lack of evidence for this practice is discussed below.

Laryngoscope Insertion and Intubation

Suctioning can traumatize the delicate mucus membranes of the newborn's oral pharynx. Chapter 7 reviewed the implications of such routine disturbances on newborn suck-swallow-breathe mechanisms. Considerably greater trauma can result from suctioning an infant delivered of a mother with meconium-stained amniotic fluid (MS). The routine in many hospitals worldwide for such MS infants is to place them on a cot or warmer separate from the mother (sometimes in another room), place a laryngoscope, and then perform deep suctioning below the vocal cords before the baby takes its first breath. This often means forceful holding of the infant's mouth open by the birth attendant or pediatric attendant in such a way that a first breath is impossible. Often MS at birth was an indication for routine separation of the baby from the mother for some hours, even if the infant seemed vigorous after this procedure.

In 2000, Wiswell and associates published the results of a large, international, multicenter trial on the effectiveness of two management routines for meconium staining.[52] Two cohorts were randomly selected from a total of 2094 vigorous infants with MS.

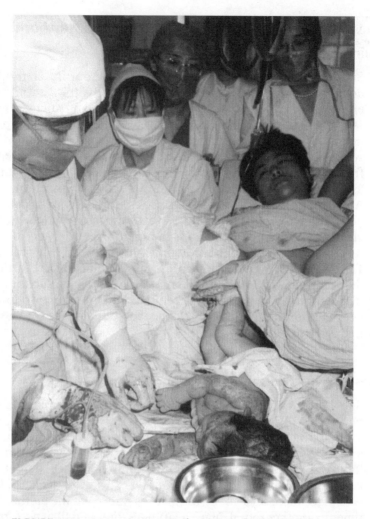

FIGURE 10-4   Meconium-stained amniotic fluid at birth has been managed with aggressive suctioning and often with insertion of laryngoscope and intubation. *Photo by Mary Kroeger, China 1997.*

One cohort received expectant management with no suctioning, and the other cohort had laryngoscopes placed, intubation, and suctioning. Results were determined by the number of infants who subsequently developed severe respiratory problems called meconium aspiration syndrome (MAS), and also by the rate of complications from the intubation/suctioning procedures themselves. Findings were that there was no statistical difference in the frequency of occurrence of MAS, with 3.2% in the intubated group and 2.7% in the expectant management group developing this complication. The authors' report 3.8% of the intubated group had "mild and transient" complications. These were bradycardia (slowed heart rate), hoarseness or stridor, laryngospasm (spasm of the throat), apnea (temporary stoppage of breathing), bleeding at the vocal cords, and cyanosis (blue color due to poor oxygenation). All of these "transient complications" can directly or indirectly affect early sucking. The conclusion from this study is that intubation and suctioning does not result in decreased incidence of meconium aspiration syndrome.

Circumcision

According to the Council on Scientific Affairs of the American Medical Association, circumcision is a non-therapeutic procedure without documented benefit for the infant.[53] Hill has raised concerns in a letter to a lactation journal about how little the matter of possible negative effects on breastfeeding from circumcision is addressed in the literature or in parental counseling.[54] Circumcision is a traumatic and painful procedure that induces hard crying and that will continue to cause postoperative pain to the newborn. Anesthetic is used in less than half of the procedures done, according to one survey.[55] This is despite the fact that the American Academy of Pediatrics (AAP) has called for the use of anesthetic.

In his letter, Hill notes 25 years of studies documenting breastfeeding difficulties in infant males who have been circumcised.[56,57] Howard et al. studied 44 infants after circumcision and found lessfrequent feeding and withdrawn, subdued, less-interactive behavior. Howard cautions that because many babies are discharged on the day the circumcision is performed, they are lost to immediate follow-up for subsequent breastfeeding problems. Breastfeeding newborns in this study required supplementation due to their mother's perception that the baby could not breastfeed or had true difficulties with feeding. Early supplementation before the onset of lactogenesis is known to be associated with breastfeeding failure. Given the strong arguments for protecting a calm, safe, pain-free environment for the newborn to transition to life outside the warmth and cushion of the uterus, Hill argues that "successful breastfeeding should be given absolute priority over neonatal circumcision." The work group on breastfeeding in the AAP has also called for avoidance of painful procedures like circumcision.[58]

Fleiss has written extensively on the initial and long-term trauma to infants from circumcision. He writes: "The radical practice of routinely circumcising babies did not begin until the Cold War era. This institutionalization of what amounted to compulsory circumcision was part of the same movement that pathologized and medicalized birth and actively discouraged breastfeeding." [59]

Routine Eye Medication, Vitamin K Injections, and Heel Sticks for Hypoglycemia Screening

In the United States, parents accept many "routines" in newborn care that seem best for the health of the newborn "just in case" there is a problem. Some of these routines interfere with early skin-to-skin contact and mother-baby interaction and they are also painful to the newborn. Discussion of the pros and cons of these various procedures is beyond the scope of this chapter, but it is hoped that the case has been made that mother-baby contact in the immediate postpartum must be a priority. The routine instillation of prophylactic eye medication to prevent eye infection (opthalmia neonatorum), the injection of Vitamin K for enhancement of immature blood clotting factors at birth, and even the routine lancing of the newborn's heel to check for hypoglycemia are all procedures for which parents need to know pros, cons, benefits, and risks, so they can give fully informed consent for allowing or declining painful procedures on their baby in the first sensitive hours right after birth.

Trauma at Birth and Later Suicide

The long-term implication for interference with the early newborn period goes beyond interference with breastfeeding and mothering. Jacobson and Bygdeman published a prospective study of birth records of 242 adults who had committed suicide by violent means who were matched with 403 biological siblings born in the same period and at the same hospitals.[60] The data extractors were blinded as to which sibling had died from violent suicide as medical charts were reviewed. A scoring system was utilized that counted traumatic birth events, including presentation other than head first (breech and other malpresentation), meconium staining, instrumental delivery, internal version, resuscitation, and other complications requiring ward care. Results showed that traumatic birth was associated with a fivefold increase in likelihood of violent suicide in men and a doubled risk in women. The authors conclude, "Minimizing pain to the infant during birth seems to be of importance in reducing the risk of violent suicide as an adult."

Crying and the Newborn

Anderson defined the concept of *mother and newborn* as "mutual caregivers" in 1976, and her research has continued to show the importance of early and sustained mother-infant contact.[61] She was a pioneer in the study of "risks of separation," and described normal crying patterns in babies. Babies continuously cared for by the parents after birth in a mutual care-giving arrangement cried only 1 minute and did not "startle" during the first hour postpartum compared with babies kept in nurseries. The latter babies (even though they had been held briefly by their mothers in the delivery room) cried 10 minutes and startled on an average of 12 times during the first hour postpartum. In a 1989 review article in which she advocates for continuous rooming-in, Anderson describes several of the dangers of prolonged crying in the newborn, including higher blood pressures, higher intracranial pressures, and less oxygen in circulating blood.[62] She argues that preventing crying and startling in a newborn may be important to the newborn's later development. Crying resembles the Valsalva maneuver (the Valsalva maneuver is an expiratory effort against a closed glottis, which increases pressure within the thoracic cavity and thereby impedes venous return of blood to the heart) in adults, and prolonged crying can obstruct venous return and can in the newborn reestablish fetal circulation in the heart during the first 4–5 days of life.[63] This danger is greatest in preterm infants, but full-term infants are also vulnerable to intracranial bleeds. In one nursery of general term newborns who appeared normal, 16 babies of 505 (3%) had hemorrhages documented on ultrasound.[64] Anderson speculated in 1989 that minimal learning disabilities could be linked to these early undetected bleeds. A later study in term, healthy infants showed a 6% incidence of intracranial hemorrhage in a cohort of 177 infants who underwent routine ultrasonography at 48 hours of age.[65] This later study tracked the cohort to 12 and 18 months and found no signs of cerebral palsy or developmental delay. Avrahami et al. report that 58 term newborns who had negative ultrasound scans were referred for further diagnosis with CT scan because they exhibited apnea, disturbances in suck and swallow, poor tone, tremors, and jerks.[66] Twenty-three of these infants subsequently underwent lumbar puncture because of evidence of intracranial

bleeds. At 14–17 months follow-up, 5 of these infants were diagnosed with psychomotor retardation. The relatively high incidence of cranial ultrasound abnormalities remains unexplained
and still of concern. Although it is not possible to connect these
adverse findings on CT scan to crying, certainly the foregoing discussion suggests that creation of a calm and supportive environment for newborns where crying is minimized is important.

Christensson and colleagues have studied the benefits of skin-
to-skin care in the first hours after normal delivery. Their primary
hypothesis in one study was that skin-to-skin contact would serve
as a soothing mechanism, resulting in less crying as the baby
transitions to extrauterine life.[67] Fifty healthy newborns were
randomly allocated to two groups of 25. One group was dried and
placed skin-to-skin prone on the mother and kept there. Group
two babies were dried, swaddled with double wrappers, and put in
a cot next to the mother. Both groups were observed for 90 minutes after delivery. The skin-to-skin group had several findings of
statistical significance: they cried less and had higher body temperatures and higher blood glucose levels at 90 minutes postpartum. The authors note that while they had expected the body
temperatures of the crying infants to increase, the reverse was
true. They also speculated that if human babies are like rat pups,
the "distress cries" of one rat pup create crying in others. They
postulate that this may occur in newborn nurseries.

This same Swedish research group has looked at the quality of
crying in the human newborn and have identified what they suggest is "genetically encoded reaction" to separation from the
mother, comparing it to the "distress call" seen in rats when pups
are separated from their mothers.[68] In one clinical trial, they found
that in a group of 29 healthy, vaginally delivered newborns, those
assigned to be kept in a cot next to the mother rather than skin-to-
skin cried 10 times more often in the first 90 minutes after delivery. Sound spectrography of the quality of the crying in this study
suggested the cry of the separated babies was a "discomfort cry."[69]

Barriers Still Exist

There are many barriers to breastfeeding, but failure to implement
Step Four of the BFHI remains a key barrier. A longitudinal mail
survey in the United States tracked women from the prenatal period
through 12 months postpartum.[70] A questionnaire survey was sent
to 1085 women who had decided during their pregnancy that they

would breastfeed. Questionnaires asked about presence or absence of five BFHI parameters: late initiation of breastfeeding, introduction of supplements, no rooming, no feeding on demand, and use of pacifiers. Only 7% of the respondents had experienced all five BFHI practices in their care. Mothers who were at the greatest risk for termination of breastfeeding had no early initiation and had supplementation of baby in the hospital (see Figure 10-5). The conclusions support that the BFHI practices are associated with a longer duration of breastfeeding and that the failure to initiate breastfeeding early is a key determinant of failure.

Rowe-Murray and Fisher in Australia conducted a prospective longitudinal study of 203 primiparous mothers to investigate the effects of mode of delivery and place of delivery (designated Baby Friendly Hospital versus non-BFH) on early mother-baby contact.[71] The study design is complex and involved a developed tool, the First Contact Index, to examine quality, quantity, and subjective experience of the first contact between mother and newborn. The sum total of these parameters were pooled to assess overall maternal emotional well-being at first contact (Figure 10-6). The tool proved to correlate well with maternal mood in the short and long term, including the retrospective rating of their experiences surrounding birth. Findings were that mothers delivered by cesarean section experienced "compromised first contact" compared with vaginally delivered mothers, whether spontaneous or instrumental mode. This finding was significant after controlling

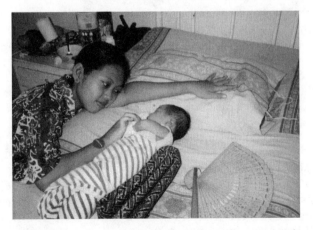

FIGURE 10-5   A first-time mother allowed unrestricted contact with her baby from birth and in the postpartum ward. West Kalimantan, Indonesia. *Photo by Mary Kroeger.*

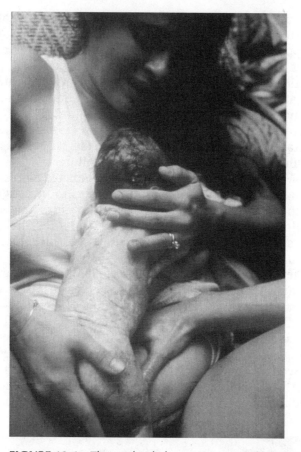

FIGURE 10-6   The mother-baby continuum. Baby leaves the womb and moves to mother's arms and body. She has the first contact and all procedures can wait for the mother and baby to learn about each other all over again—from the outside. *Photo © Harriette Hartigan.*

for other variables, including birth weight and newborn asphyxia. Among the four hospitals included in this study, the designated BFHI hospital had significantly more mothers scoring high on the Index regardless of mode of delivery, although cesarean-delivered mothers still had lower ratings than vaginally delivered mothers. The authors conclude that cesarean section, even in a BFHI setting, still has a negative impact on early mother-baby interaction (see Chapter 8). They conclude that there continue to be deficiencies in maternity care in regards to ensuring early optimal contact between mother and baby, and their discussion emphasizes that in addition to impact on short-term and long-term mothering, they warn against the negative impact of separation on the baby.

In light of evidence of sophisticated perceptual capacities in the newborn and that early experiences help organize the developing infant's brain, denial of the opportunity to exercise inborn behaviors may have as yet unidentified, adverse consequences for development.[72] In addition, since the mother so clearly frames the infant's social world, it is plain that her emotional state will be of importance to the infant's optimal development even at this early stage of life. Practices that optimize her well-being are likely to have consequences for both of them.

With the rapidly rising cesarean section rates in many countries, including Australia, these findings are of concern. Immediate skin-to-skin contact, although not impossible after cesarean section, is certainly difficult due to the surgical set-up with sterile drapes and the fact that the mother is supine and has both arms restricted by monitors and/or intravenous lines. In China, there has been a concerted effort in BFHI hospitals to ensure some cheek-to-cheek contact and "gazing" time (see Figure 10-7). In the United States it is usually the father of the baby who is the first to hold and snuggle a cesarean section–born infant. This is certainly an excellent alternative to the baby being put in a nursery, but it may allow for additional rationalizing that early mother-baby contact can wait. The cesarean section may have been planned or an emergency. If it was an emergency and there are adverse outcomes, early contact may be compromised.

A Guide to Effective Care in Pregnancy and Childbirth[50] has a section that highlights results of Cochrane reviews spanning 30 years of research on separation of mother and baby in hospitals postpartum.[73] Randomized controlled trials on restriction of contact in the early hours versus immediate and prolonged contact showed association with maternal affectionate behavior "was significantly less evident among mothers whose contact had been restricted than among mothers whose care encouraged liberal contact." With contact after the immediate postpartum period (that is rooming-in versus non-rooming-in), there was "association with less affectionate maternal behavior and more frequent feelings of incompetence and lack of confidence" among mothers who had had restricted contact. One well-conducted study in the review showed that routine separation of mothers from their babies in the hospital led to subsequent risk of child abuse and neglect among socially deprived, first-time mothers.

Barriers to early, sustained mother-baby contact are also present in a developing countries. Even where there is a predominance

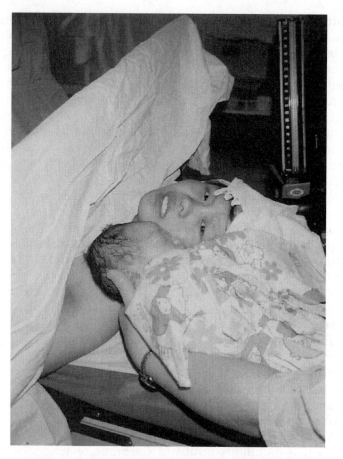

FIGURE 10-7   Mother undergoing cesarean section has brief cheek-to-cheek contact and gazing time. Her hands are restrained. *Photo by Mary Kroeger, China 1997.*

of homebirths, the hospital culture can quickly adopt routines that are not supportive of early initiation. In Cambodia, during midwife refresher training, maternity staff often resist trying early skin-to-skin contact, stating "our mothers are too tired," This new practice had to be demonstrated and most of the time mother were found to be happy to hold their newborns[74] (Figure 10-8). In Malawi, when maternity staff at one hospital saw the Swedish video *Delivery Self-Attachment,* they said, "Only Swedish babies crawl up the mother like that, not African babies." Less than two hours later, work in the busy maternity ward provided the midwives a chance to see that indeed Malawian babies self-attach as well.

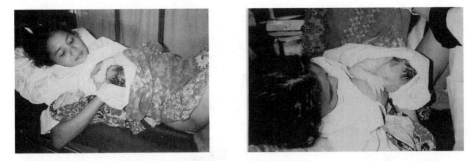

FIGURES 10-8   This Cambodian mother was used to having the baby taken to the family after delivery. The immediate skin-to-skin routine introduced during midwife refresher training showed staff that she was not "too tired" to hold and suckle her baby. *Photo by Mary Kroeger, 1999.*

Protecting the Mother-Baby Continuum

Mothering a newborn is a complex behavior that is affected by social, cultural, physiological, and environmental factors, many of which precede the labor and delivery events. Previous chapters outlined specific labor and delivery interventions that can enhance or detract from a woman's immediate ability to assume mothering and initiated breastfeeding. An immediate postpartum environment created by a calmed baby put immediately skin-to-skin with the mother sets in motion a cascade of hormones: oxytocin, prolactin, beta-endorphins, and a host of other neuroendocrine factors. Even after a long and difficult childbirth, a woman will cuddle and gaze at her baby and engage in loving exploration if she is protected and supported. This behavior is "programmed" genetically to ensure a continuum after delivery that has encouraged the survival of our species.

Summary Points for Protecting the Mother-Baby Continuum

- Evidence shows that early skin-to-skin contact between mother and newborn is the physiologic norm.
- A baby left on its mother's abdomen has inborn behaviors that lead the baby to the breast to feed.
- Step Four of the BFHI Ten Steps to Successful Breastfeeding states, "Help mothers initiate breast-feeding within half-hour of birth."
- Evidence shows that routines and interventions during childbirth and immediately after birth can interfere with bonding, mothering, and optimal initiation of breastfeeding.

• Kangaroo care (skin-to-skin) for premature infants stabilizes temperature, heart rate, respiratory rate, blood sugar, reduces crying, encourages deeper sleep, supports breastfeeding, and reassures new mothers

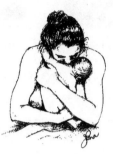

References

1. WHO/UNICEF (Joint Statement). 1989. *Protecting, Promoting, and Supporting Breast-Feeding: The Special Role of Maternity Services.* Geneva: WHO.
2. WHO. 1998. *Evidence for the Ten Steps to Successful Breast-feeding.* Geneva: WHO/CHD/98.9.
3. Righard L, Alade MO. 1990. Effect of delivery room routines on success of first breast-feed. *Lancet* 336:1105–1107.
4. Ransjo-Arvidson A, Matthieson, Gunilla L, et al. 2001. Maternal analgesia during labor disturbs newborn behavior: Effects on breastfeeding, temperature, and crying. *Birth* 28(1):5–12.
5. Matthieson A, Ransjo-Arvidson A, Gunilla L, et al. 2001. Postpartum maternal oxytocin release by newborns: Effects of infant hand massage and suckling. *Birth* 28(1):13–19.
6. Lagercrantz H, Slotkin TA. 1986. The stress of being born. *Scientific American* 254:91–102.
7. Nissan E, Lilja G, Matthiesen AS, et al. 1996. Effects of maternal pethidine on infants' developing breastfeeding behavior. *Research* 4(2):73–78.
8. Varendi H, Porter RH, Winberg J. 1994. Does the newborn find the nipple by smell? *Lancet* 344(8928):989–990.
9. Varendi H, Porter R. 2001. Breast odour as the only maternal stimulus elicits crawling toward the odour source. *Acta Paediatr* 90(4):372–375.

10. Newton N. 1971. Trebly sensuous woman. *Psychology Today* 71(July):68–71.
11. Hofmeyr GJ, Nikodem VC, Wolman W, et al. 1991. Companionship to modify the clinical birth environment: Effects on progress and perception of labour, and breastfeeding. *Brit J of Obstet Gynecol* 98:756–764.
12. Klaus M, Kennel J, Klaus PH. 1993. *Mothering the Mother.* Reading, MA: Addison Wesley Publishing.
13. Odent M. 1992. Colostrum and civilization. A chapter in: *The Nature of Birth and Breast-feeding.* London: Bergin and Garvey.
14. Kitzinger S. 1995. Commentary. Breastfeeding: Biocultural perspectives. In: Stuart-Macadam P, and Dettwyler KA (Eds.). *Breastfeeding: Biocultural Perspectives.* New York: Aldine De Gruyter.
15. Sugarman M. 1977. Paranatal [SIC] Influences on Maternal-Infant Attachment. Presentation at a seminar on development of infants and parents, Emmanuel College, Boston, October 1976. Reprinted in *Amer J Orthopsychiat* 47(3):407–421.
16. WHO/UNICEF. 1992. *Global Criteria for the Baby Friendly Hospital Initiative.* Geneva and New York: WHO/UNICEF.
17. Armstrong, H. 2003. Personal communication.
18. UNICEF. 1998. *Reassessment of Baby-Friendly Hospitals and Maternity Services: A Guide to Developing a National Process. Part VII.* pp. 3–5. New York: UNICEF Programme Division.
19. Lazarov M. 1994. *Barriers and Solutions to the Global Ten Steps to Successful Breastfeeding: A summary of in-depth interviews with Hospitals participating in the WHO-UNICEF Baby-Friendly Hospital Initiative Interim Program in the United States United States.* Committee for UNICEF. April 1994. New York: UNICEF.
20. Kroeger M. 1996–2001. In: *Trip Reports to American College of Nurse Midwives for Life Savings Skills Training Activities* in West Kalimantan, Indonesia - April 1996; Jakarta, Indonesia–July 1996; Battambang, Cambodia–February 1999; Phnom Penh, Cambodia–August 2001. Unpublished. On file at American College of Nurse-Midwives. Washington DC.
21. Heiser B. 2003. Personal communication.
22. Lazarov M. 2003. Personal communication.
23. Righard L, Alade MO. 1990. Effect of delivery room routines on success of first breast-feed. *Lancet* 336:1105–1107.
24. Widstrom AM, Wahlberg AS, Matthiesen P, et al. 1990. Short-term effects of early suckling and touch of the nipple on maternal behavior. *Early Hum Dev* 21:153–163.
25. Bullough CHW, Msuku R, Karonda L. 1989. Early suckling and postpartum haemorrhage: Controlled by trial in deliveries by traditional birth attendants. *Lancet* 2:522–525.
26. International Lactation Consultant Association. 1999. *Evidenced-Based Guidelines for Breastfeeding Management during the First*

Fourteen Days. Funded by United States Maternal and Child Health Bureau, April 1999.

27. Armstrong H. 2003. Personal communication.

28. UNICEF. 1998. *Reassessment of Baby-Friendly Hospitals and Maternity Services: A Guide to Developing a National Process. Part VII.* pp. 3–5. New York: UNICEF Programme Division.

29. De Chateau P, Holmberg H, Jakobsson K, et al. 1977. A study of factors promoting and inhibiting lactation. *Develop Med Child Neurol* 19:575–584.

30. Righard L, Alade MO. 1990. Effect of delivery room routines on success of first breast-feed. *Lancet* 336:1105–1107.

31. Widstrom AM, Wahlberg AS, Matthiesen P, et al. 1990. Short-term effects of early suckling and touch of the nipple on maternal behavior. *Early Hum Dev* 21:153–163.

32. Klaus M. 1998. Mother and infant: Early emotional ties. *Pediatrics* 102(5):1244–1246.

33. Uvnas-Moberg K. 1989. The gastrointestinal tract in growth and reproduction. *Sci Am* 261(1):78–83.

34. Marchini G, Linden A. 1992. Cholecystokinin, a satiety signal in newborn infants? *J Dev Physiol* 17(5):215–219.

35. Hoover K. 1994. Handout. "That Sleepy Child." In: Hoover, K. 2002. An 18-hour Breastfeeding Class for Maternal and Child Healthcare Professionals. Philadelphia: Department of Health.

36. Varendi H, Porter RH, Winberg J. 1994. Does the newborn find the nipple by smell? *Lancet* 344(8928):989–990.

37. Varendi H, Porter R. 2001. Breast odour as the only maternal stimulus elicits crawling toward the odour source. *Acta Paediatr* 90(4):372–375.

38. Rey ES, Martinez HG. 1983. Rational de Ninio Prematuro; Manejo: Proceedings of the conferences I Cursi de Medicina Fetal y Neonatal, held Bogota, Columbia, March 17-19, 1983, pp. 137–151 (Spanish).

39. Anderson GC. 1991. Current knowledge about skin-to-skin (kangaroo) care for pre-term infants. *J Perinatol* 11(3):216–226.

40. Hadeed AJ, Ludington-Hoe SM, Siegal C. 1995. Skin-to-skin contact (SSC) between mother and infant reduces idiopathic apnea of prematurity. *Ped Res* 37(94) part 2:280A; Abstract #1233.

41. Karlsson H. 1996. Skin-to-skin care: Heat balance. *Arc Dis Childhood* 75 F: 130–132.

42. Anderson GC, Chiu S-H, Morrison B, et al. (in press). Skin-to-skin for breastfeeding difficulties postbirth. In: Tiffany Field (Ed.), *Advances in Touch.* New Brunswick, NJ: Johnson & Johnson.

43. Ludington-Hoe SM, Anderson GC, Simpson S, et al. 1999. Birth-related fatigue in 34-36 week pre-term neonates: Rapid recovery with very early kangaroo (skin-to-skin) care. *JOGNN* 26(1):94–103.

44. Feldman R, Weller A, Sirota L, et al. 2002. Skin-to-skin (Kangaroo care) promotes self-regulation in premature infants: Sleep-wake cyclicity, arousal modulation, and sustained exploration. *Dev Psychol* 38 (2):194–207.

45. Hurst NM, Valentine CJ, Renfro L, et al. 1997. Skin-to-skin holding in the neonatal intensive care unit influences maternal milk volume. *J Perinatol* 17(3):213–217.

46. Ludington-Hoe SM, Swinth JY. 1996. Developmental aspects of Kangaroo Care. *JOGNN* 25(8):691–703.

47. Carbajal R, Veerapen S, Couderic S, et al. 2003. Analgesic effect of breastfeeding in term neonates: Randomized controlled trial. *BM J* 326: (7379):13.

48. Colson SD, Rooy L, Hawdon JM. 2003. Biological nurturing increases duration of breastfeeding for a vulnerable cohort. *MIDIRS Midwifery Digest* 13(1):92–97.

49. WHO, UNFPA, UNICEF, World Bank. 2000. *Managing Complications in Pregnancy and Childbirth: A Guide for Midwives and Doctors.* Geneva: World Health Organization. Department of Reproductive Health and Research C-59.

50. Enkin M, Keirse M, Renfrew M, et al. 2000. *A Guide to Effective Care in Pregnancy and Childbirth,* 3rd ed. Oxford: Oxford University Press.

51. Gilstrip LC, Oh W (Eds). 2002. *Guidelines for Perinatal Care,* 5th ed. Jointly published by the American College of Obstetrics and Gynecology and the American Academy of Pediatrics.

52. Wiswell T, Gannon CM, Jacob J, et al. 2000. Delivery room management of the apparently vigorous meconium-stained neonate: Results of a multicenter, international collaborative trial. *Pediatrics* 105(1):1–7.

53. American Medical Association, Council on Scientific Affairs. 1999. Report 10: *Neonatal Circumcision.* Chicago IL: American Medical Association.

54. Hill G. 2003. Breastfeeding must be given priority over circumcision. Letter in *J Human Lact* 19 (1):21.

55. Stang HJ, Snellman LW. 1998. Circumcision practice patterns in the United States. *Pediatrics* 101:e5.

56. Marshall RE, Porter FL, Rogers AG, et al. 1982. Circumcision II: Effects on mother-infant interaction. *Early Hum Dev* 7:367–374.

57. Howard CR, Howard FM, Weitzman ML. 1994. Acetaminophen analgesia in neonatal circumcision: The effect of pain. *Pediatrics* 93:641–646.

58. Academy of Pediatrics, Workgroup on Breastfeeding. 1997. Breastfeeding and the use of human milk. *Pediatrics* 100:1035–1039.

59. Fleiss P. 1997. The case against circumcision. *Mothering Magazine* Winter 1997:36–45.

60. Jacobson B, Bygdeman M. 1998. Obstetric care and proneness of offspring to suicide as adults: Case-control study. *BMJ* 317: 1347–1349.
61. Anderson GC. 1977. The mother and her newborn: Mutual care-givers. *J Obstet, Gynecol Neonatal Nurs* 6(5):50–57.
62. Anderson GC.1989. Risk in mother-infant separation post birth. *IMAGE: Journal of Nursing Scholarship* 21(4):196–199.
63. Lind J, Stern L, Wegelius C. 1964. Human and fetal circulation. Republished in: Walsh SZ, WW Meyer WW, Lind J (Eds.). *The Human Fetal and Neonatal Circulation* (pp. 89–94). Springfield, IL: Thomas, 1974.
64. Hayden CK, Shadduck KE, Richardson CV, et al., 1985. Subependymal germal matrix hemorrhage in full-term neonates. *Pediatrics* 75:714–718.
65. Haataja L, Mercuri E, Cowan F, et al. 2000. Cranial ultrasound abnormalities in full term infants in a postnatal ward: outcome at 12 and 18 months. *Arch Dis Child Fetal Neonatal Ed* 82(2):F128–33.
66. Avrahami E, Amzel S, Katz R, et al. 1996. CT demonstration of intracranial bleeding in term newborns with mild clinical symptoms. *Clin Radiol* 51:31–34.
67. Christensson K, Siles C, Moreno L, et al. 1992. Temperature, metabolic adaptation and crying in healthy full-term newborns cared for skin-to-skin or in a cot. *Acta Paediatr* 81:488–493.
68. Christensson K, Cabrera T, Christensson E, et al. 1995. Separation calling the human neonate in the absence of maternal body contact. *Acta Paediatr* 84(5):468–473.
69. Michelsson K, Christensson K, Rothganger H, et al. 1996. Crying in separated and non-separated newborns: Sound spectrographc analysis. *Acta Paediatr* 85(4):471–475.
70. DiGirolamo AM, Laurence M, Grummer-Strawn L, et al. 2001. Maternity care practices: Implications for breastfeeding. *Birth* 28(2):94–100.
71. Rowe-Murray H, Fisher J. 2001. Operative intervention in delivery is associated with compromised early mother-infant interaction. *Brit J Obstet Gynaecol* 108:1068–1075.
72. Kjellmer I, Winberg J. 1994. The neurobiology of parent-infant interaction in the newborn: An introduction. *Acta Paediatr* 397(Suppl):71–76.
73. Thompson M, Westreich R. 2000. Restriction of mother-infant contact in the immediate post-natal period. In: Enkin M, Keirse M, Neilson J, et al. *A Guide to Effective Care in Pregnancy and Childbirth*, 3rd ed. Oxford: Oxford University Press, 429–430.
74. Kroeger M, Thomas W. 1999. *Trip Report to American College of Nurse Midwives for Life Savings Skills Training*. Battambang, Cambodia - February. Unpublished. On file at ACNM, Washington, DC.

CHAPTER 11

MATERNAL BLEEDING POSTPARTUM AND BREASTFEEDING

"Postpartum hemorrhage...is the most important single cause of maternal death in the world; it is estimated to claim 150,000 maternal lives annually, mainly in developing countries."

World Health Organization, 1994

Postpartum Bleeding and Early Breastfeeding

The mother-baby continuum serves the mother as much as the newborn, and early initation of breastfeeding has benefits for the mother that are often not appreciated. Labbok, who has written about the long-term benefits of breastfeeding, reminds us that breastfeeding is sometimes called the final stage of labor.[1] After a normal delivery, uterine contractions, stimulated by oxytocin, continue to reduce the area of attachment of the placenta to the uterine wall and force separation of the placenta, allowing it to drop into the lower part of the uterus. Contractions then expel the placenta, cord, and attached membranes, in a process technically called the third stage of labor. Prevention of life-threatening bleeding from the open "wound" where the placenta was attached is accomplished by continued oxytocin pulsation, causing uterine contractions that compress the vascular site of attachment and minimize blood loss. When, for a variety of reasons, this mechanism does not function properly, heavy bleeding and eventually life-threatening postpartum hemorrhage can result.

Hemorrhage is a major cause of maternal mortality worldwide, and additonal study has shown that the majority of these deaths occur in the first four hours after birth, in association with the delivery of the placenta or soon after[2,3] (Figure 11-1). Safe Motherhood programs recommend a set of interventions to pre-

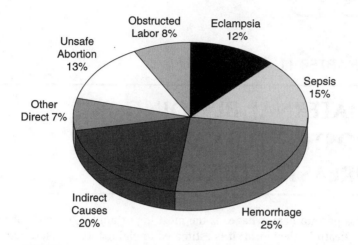

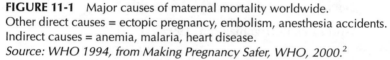

FIGURE 11-1   Major causes of maternal mortality worldwide.
Other direct causes = ectopic pregnancy, embolism, anesthesia accidents.
Indirect causes = anemia, malaria, heart disease.
Source: WHO 1994, from Making Pregnancy Safer, WHO, 2000.[2]

vent and treat postpartum bleeding and while not foremost among them, early breastfeeding is recognized as one intervention to facilitate placental delivery and help prevent excessive bleeding.[4-6] Although this practice is founded on empiric observation and clinical common sense, it has never been demonstarted in a rigorous research study.

One Randomized Controlled Trial

To the knowledge of the author, only one study has investigated the connection between breastfeeding and postpartum blood loss. A large, randomized controlled trial in Malawi of over 4200 home deliveries studied the role of early skin-to-skin contact and initiation of breastfeeding and subsequent impact on postpartum bleeding.[7] Traditional birth attendants (TBAs) were divided into two groups. One group (n = 23) was taught to deliver the placenta physiologically, to put the baby immediately on the mother's abdomen and then encourage immediate breastfeeding. The control group (n = 26) continued with the traditional care, which in this setting called for the baby to be cared for immediately after birth by relatives and letting the mother rest. TBAs in both groups were taught to estimate the amount of blood loss. Several checks for inaccurate reporting were built into the study and the study group of TBAs were not aware that

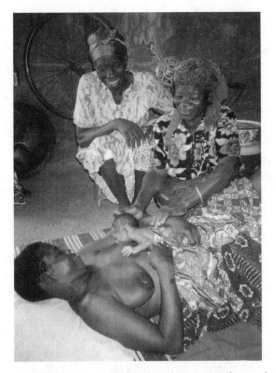

FIGURE 11-2 Traditional midwives can learn about the importance of colostrum and the life-saving effects of early initiation. *Photo by Mary Kroeger, Ghana, 2000.*

the early breastfeeding intervention was hypothesized to impact postpartum bleeding (Figure 11-2). Findings were that there was no statistical difference in postpartum blood loss between the early breastfeeding and the control groups. A concurrent hospital trial with a similar population of mothers was conducted to test the premise that newborns can successfully suckle immediately after birth. Nurse-midwives conducted 76 deliveries and found that 20 of the newborns suckled within 5 mins, 53 suckled within 10 mins, and all were suckling by 20 minutes after delivery. Because the majority of newborns in this substudy began suckling after the placenta had separated, authors argue that the early suckling could not be associated with delivery of the placenta. Their discussion points out that a significant finding in the smaller trial was that all babies were suckling by 20 minutes postpartum, with the mean being 7.25 minutes. The authors also suggest that if the larger trial had been done with literate and numerate nurse-midwives, the possibility of inaccurate estimation of blood loss might be eliminated, and they urge additional study.

This study has not been replicated, although two later studies shed some additional light. Bullough's group studied the effects of nipple stimulation in the third stage of labor on blood loss in a very small randomized controlled trial.[8] After delivery, but before the delivery of the placenta, three groups of mothers underwent differing management regimes. Group one mothers (n = 6) were taught to compress their nipples in an action mimicking sucking for 15 minutes; group two (n =3) was administered Syntometrine injection, a medication combining both oxytocin and Ergotmetrine and known to cause uterine contraction and to reduce bleeding; group three (n = 5) was the control, with physiologic management of third stage and no special action taken. The placenta, still undelivered, was used as an "in situ hydrostatic bag," and after delivery the umbilical cord extending from the maternal vagina was cannulated with an internal pressure catheter. Authors note that previous study established this technicque as accurate for assessing intrauterine pressure. Results demonstrated that nipple stimulation produced a significant rise in uterine pressure compared to the controls. Pressure in the study group was also higher than the Syntometrine group, but not significantly. Blood loss was least in the syntometrine group (mean = 83 ml), but the nipple stimulation group lost considerably less blood (mean = 166 ml) compared to the control group (mean = 257 ml). The authors conclude that in resource-poor settings where syntometrine and other uterine contractor medicines are not available, nipple stimulation is an effective way to reduce postpartum bleeding. The authors do not explain why they did not use another study group of mothers who put their babies skin-to-skin with support to breastfeed.

Chua and associates in Singapore measured the effects of breastfeeding and nipple stimulation on postpartum uterine activity.[9] Eleven mothers in active labor at term, who had had no labor interventions or medication, completed spontaneous vaginal delivery of their babies and placentas and then received no postpartum prophylactic medicines to encourage uterine contractions. Immediately after third stage, a pressure transducer was inserted into the uterus to measure and record postpartum uterine contractions for 30 minutes. Thirty minutes after delivery, each mother, "acting as her own control," stated her feeding choice. The six mothers who opted not to breastfeed were asked to manually stimulate one nipple for the next 30 minutes while uterine activity was recorded. Five mothers elected to breastfeed, and the article states that at 30 minutes after placement of the pressure transducer "the baby was then put to breast." The authors had previously established the natural decline in uterine activity over time in the first 90 minutes postpartum. Findings were that there was a median increase in uterine activity of 93% from baseline in the breastfeeding group and 66% in the nipple stimulation group, respectively. The authors note that this is a "marked increase" considering a natural decline in uterine activity in the first 90 minutes of 30% of the initial immedate postpartum value. A weakness of the study is that there is no discussion of the individual variation among the five mother-baby pairs in regards to time of first effective latch-on or duration of the breastfeeding during the 30 minutes of recording. The study concludes that both breastfeeding and nipple stimualtion increase uterine activity, with breastfeeding being the more effective method. Postpartum blood loss was not measured in this study.

The three research studies reviewed in the preceding paragraphs do not provide much evidence to support breastfeeding as an intervention to reduce blood loss. The large, randomized trial had results suggesting that breastfeeding is not an effective strategy to reduce blood loss, but there was considerable reason to question the accuracy of measurements made by nonnumerate traditional midwives. The other two studies had conclusive

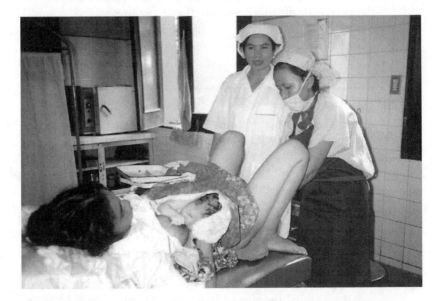

FIGURE 11-3 Midwives in Cambodia manage third stage by giving oxytocin injection after the baby is delivered, and then observing closely for signs of separation from the uterine wall before attempting to deliver the placenta. The baby is dried well, placed skin-to-skin on the mother, covered with dry cloth, and then encouraged to have contact with the mother's nipples. *Photo by Mary Kroeger, ACNM LSS © Training, 1999.*

results, but extremely small sample sizes. All three studies concluded there is a need for further research, because in spite of global recommendations that oxytocic medications be available in all facilites, including the first-line referral centers, these medicines are not always available in district hospitals in resource-poor countries, nor are they available to most traditional home birth attendants.[6]

Chapter 8 discussed a study in which maternal plasma levels of oxytocin and prolactin where sampled at 2 days postpartum in 20 vaginally delivered mothers compared to 17 mothers delivered by cesarean section. Findings were that significantly more oxytocin pulses occurred in the vaginally delivered mothers compared with those who were surgically delivered.[10] The number of oxytocin pulses was correlated to duration of exclusive breastfeeding in the vaginal delivery group and vaginal delivery seems to foster earlier, more effective secretion of both oxytocin and prolactin. These findings suggest that breastfeeding is correlated with control of bleeding well into the early postpartum, even after the potential dangers of the first 4 hours after delivery. During the four to six weeks after delivery, the mother's uterus gradually returns to prepregnant size and the bleeding from the placental site diminishes and stops. This happens for all mothers, whether they breastfeed or not. However, breastfeeding, with the continued pulsitile secretion of oxytocin that results, likely plays a significant role in this process.

Prophylactic Oxytocics for Bleeding and Breastfeeding

Little is known about the impact of routine use of prophylactic oxytocic medications on breastfeeding outcomes. In an unpublished literature review, Steel examined research on the ergot derivative medications (Ergometrine and Methergine), on synthetic oxytocin medications (Syntocinon, Pitocin), and also on Syntometrine, a combination of the two types of medications.[11] At the time the paper was written, the use of prostaglandins for control of postpartum bleeding was not common and this class of medications was not reviewed. Steel's article reviews a number of studies on the ergot alkaloids and their effect on prolactin levels. One study was on twelve nonbreastfeeding mothers at three days postpartum of measured baseline prolactin levels, and then levels at intervals over the next 150 minutes after administration of a standard dose of 0.2 mg of IV Ergometrine.[12] Results showed a marked lowering of the serum prolactin, especially in the 1–2 hours after administration. Another study reported significant lowering of serum prolactin in ten nonbreastfeeding mothers receiving 0.2 mg of oral ergometrine three times a day for seven days.[13] Levels were compared to six postpartum nonlactating mothers who received no drug. Seven of the ten mothers still had clear evidence of milk secretion (breast engorgement and pain) but three had "progressive lactation inhibition." Two mothers in the same study who were breastfeeding were given IV Ergometrine and one of the two also had oral ergometrine. This second lactating mother failed to show a rise in prolactin in response to suckling. These authors conclude that routine use of ergometrine may suppress milk production.

In another study, a different ergot preparation, Methergine, was given as an injection of 0.2 mg to 14 nonbreastfeeding mothers after delivery of the placenta.[14] Controls (15) were given normal saline injections. Results showed a "dampening" of the rise in prolactin levels in the study group compared with the controls.

A final study was a subset of a randomized controlled trial on the use of different methods to manage the third stage of labor.[15] One of the management protocols tested was use of Ergometrine combined with physiologic management of delivery of the placenta. In the subset of 168 women, each group investigated the possible effects of Ergometrine on serum prolactin levels and the duration of breastfeeding. No difference was found in serum prolactin levels at 48 and 72 hours postpartum. However, women who had not received the drug were more likely to continue breastfeeding. In the first week after birth, 15% of the Ergometrine group had stopped breastfeeding compared with 7% of the group with no Ergometrine. The most common reason given by the Ergometrine group was "hungry baby, insufficient milk" (77%) compared with 47% of the nonmedicated group giving this reason. More mothers in the Ergometrine group had stopped breastfeeding at 6 weeks postpartum compared with the non-Ergometrine group. The author concludes that Ergometrine should not be given to women routinely if they plan to breastfeed. The Steel review cites no references on oxytocin use for control of bleeding and impact on breastfeeding, but does cite two studies that showed that the administration of exogenous oxytocin does not inhibit let-down and that oxytocin in nasal spray in fact has been used to enhance breast milk let-down.

Oxytocin is the standard medication given prophylactically to prevent postpartum bleeding in the United States, and is increasingly available for prevention and treatment of postpartum bleeding worldwide. However, Ergometrine is still widely used in many countries, and in at least some countries oral Ergometrine is routinely administered three times a day to all mothers in the postnatal wards.[18]

Conclusions

Given the evidence that ergot derivatives may interfere with pro-lactin secretion and with breastfeeding duration, it should not be given as a routine, but rather as a life-saving medication when postpartum bleeding is not controlled by oxytocin (See Box 11-1).

Box 11-1   Routine Ergometrine May Interfere with Early Breastfeeding

Eva Middleton was the executive Director of the Belize non-governmental organization, the Breast Is Best League (BIB) for 12 years, from 1982 to 1994. The BIB League promoted early and exclusive breastfeeding nationally and trained health workers and community volunteers in breastfeeding support in this small Central American country. Eva delivered all five of her children normally at the government hospital in Belize City and had no history of unusual postpartum bleeding. Eva recalls:

> Right after the delivery and again in the postnatal ward I was always given ergometrine tablets to take several times a day. These pills caused severe cramping and after the

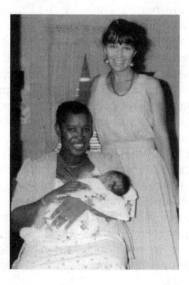

FIGURE 11-4 Eva Middleton recalls that routine ergometrine postpartum may have interfered with early breast-feeding. It is still being routinely given in government hospitals in Belize. *Left to right:* Eva, infant daughter Rhonda, and author in Belize, 1986. *Photo used with permission.*

delivery of my fifth child the pain was so severe I am ashamed to say that I dreaded putting little Rhonda to breast. The contractions of my uterus with the breastfeeding coupled with the tablets was almost too much to bear. I think some women avoided breastfeeding at the hospital while they were getting those pills and it interfered with getting off to a good start.[19]

Summary Points for Protecting the Mother-Baby Continuum

- One large, randomized controlled trial has been inconclusive about the role of early breastfeeding as a means of reducing postpartum blood loss.
- Breastfeeding, nipple stimulation, and skin-to-skin contact all stimulate oxytocin production in the mother and are likely to play a role in reducing postpartum bleeding.
- Limited research suggests a negative association between Ergometrine given to the mother postpartum and duration of breastfeeding. Alternative oxytocics should be used as the first line of prevention and control of hemorrhage whenever possible.
- More research is needed to document the role of early immediate breastfeeding in reducing postpartum bleeding.

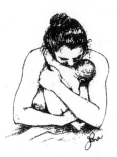

References

1. Labbok M. 1999. Health sequelae of breastfeeding for the mother. *ClinPerinatol*, 26(2):491–503.
2. WHO. 2000. *Making Pregnancy Safer: Report by the Secretariat.* December 5, 2000. In: Annex: Maternal Deaths – Main Causes and Interventions. Geneva: WHO.

3. Kane TT, El-Kady AA, Saleh S, et al. 1992. Maternal mortality in Giza, Egypt: Magnitude, causes, and prevention. *Stud Fam Planning*, 23:45–57.

4. Marshall MA, Buffington ST. 1998. *Life Savings Skills Manual for Midwives*. 3 ed. Module 5: Prevention and Treatment of Hemorrhage. Washington, DC: American College of Nurse-Midwives.

5. Klein S. 1995. *A Book for Midwives: A Manual for Traditional Birth Attendants and Community Midwives*. Palo Alto, Calif: The Hesperian Foundation.

6. WHO. 1994. *Mother-Baby Package: Implementing Safe Motherhood in Countries*. WHO/FHE/MSM/94.11. Geneva: WHO.

7. Bullough CHW, Msuku R, Karonda L. 1989. Early suckling and postpartum haemorrhage: Controlled by trial in deliveries by traditional birth attendants. *Lancet*, 2: 522–525.

8. Irons DW, Sriskandabalan P, Bullough CHW. 1994. A simple alternative to parenteral oxytocics for the third stage of labor. *Int Fed Gynecol & Obstet*, 46:15–18.

9. Chua S, Arulkumarin S, Lim I, et al. 1994. Influence of breastfeeding and nipple stimulation on postpartum uterine activity. *Br J of Obstet and Gynaecol*, 101:804–805.

10. Nissen E, Uvnas-Moberg K, Svensson K, et al. 1996. Different patterns of oxytocin prolactin but not cortisol release during breastfeeding in women delivered by cesarean section or by the vaginal route. *Early Hum Dev*, 45:103–118

11. Steel A. 1993. Routine use of oxytocics and their effect on breastfeeding. Unpublished. Wellstart International, Expanded Program of Breastfeeding. Supported by USAID Cooperative Agreement No. 5966-A-00-1045-00.

12. Shane JM, Naftoklin JM. 1974. Effect of ergonovine maleate on puerperal prolactin. *Am J Obstet Gynecol*, 120:129–131.

13. Canales ES, Garrido JT, Zarate A, et al. 1975. Effect of ergonovine on prolactin secretion on milk let-down. *Obstet Gynecol*, 48(2): 228–229.

14. Weiss G, Klein S, Shenkman L, et al. 1975. Effect of methylerogonovine on puerperal prolactin secretion. *Obstet Gyncol* 46(2):209–210.

15. Begley CM. 1990. The effect of ergometrine on breast feeding. *Midwifery*, 6:60–72.

16. Luhman L. 1993. The effect of intranasal oxytocin on lactation. *Am J Obstet Gynecol*, 21:713–717.

17. Ruis H, Rolland R, Doesburg W, et al. 1981. Oxytocin enhances onset of lactation among mothers delivering prematurely. *Br Med Journal*, 283:340–342.

18. McKenzie D. 2003. Personal communication in regards to postpartum protocol from MCH Unit, Ministry of Health, Belize.

19. Middleton E. 2003. Personal communication.

CHAPTER 12

RESTORING THE CONTINUUM

"Healing begins at the moment of birth—the unity of the mother and babe is maintained as she receives into her arms the fruit of her labor and loving... in western culture, the tearing apart of this primary unit is the first step in a series of rituals which are, in fact, the opposite of healing."

Jeannine Parvati-Baker, midwife and author, 1974

Childbirth and Breastfeeding in the New Millennium

Breastfeeding begins on the "other side of childbirth." Childbirth educators, birth attendants, and breastfeeding care providers must embrace and act on the evidence. While sometimes necessary, pain medications, other interventions in labor, and surgical delivery have both early and extended effects on the newborn and breastfeeding. Mothers and families need to know that the benefits of normal labor physiology (complete with all the intensity that labor brings) and of normal unassisted delivery (with the strenuous effort and the incredible empowerment of pushing out one's baby) are significant. As a result of a truly normal childbirth process, both mother and newborn are hormonally "programmed" with beta-endorphins, catacholamines, and physiologic levels of oxytocin to transition together beyond the birth. As the new century begins, changes in medical technology, medical training, and medical research have had profound effects on pregnancy, childbirth, newborn care, and infant feeding. This book has focused on the events and interventions surrounding childbirth and breastfeeding, but it is useful to reflect on the beginning of the partnership: pregnancy. A mother's link with her unborn child begins at conception and grows with the pregnancy; her hopes, worries, and anticipation about becoming a mother often intensify as the baby grows inside her.

Modern technology has introduced a whole new dimension in screening procedures in the prenatal period. Ultrasonography, rare 30 years ago, is now the norm rather than the exception for all pregnant women in the United States. Many pregnant women have multiple scans and parents may routinely learn the gender of the fetus and even receive sonogram "pictures" or a videotape of their unborn baby. Prenatal testing for genetic and other developmental and metabolic disorders has become the expected standard of care in industrialized countries and, where legal, families may terminate the pregnancy if the developing fetus is seriously abnormal. The relatively new specialty of maternal-fetal medicine provides care of the fetus even in newly diagnosed pregnancies. Intrauterine surgery to correct fetal abnormalities brings hope to parents who long for a normal newborn, yet it subjects the developing baby to procedures that are probably painful and may have additional effects that are as yet unknown. The field of infertility diagnosis and treatment has grown tremendously, and a host of medicines and procedures now allow infertile couples, who in the past might never have conceived, to plan and carry a baby to term. *In vitro* fertilization, along with the various alternatives to timing of harvesting and implanting embryos, now enjoys increasing success and often produces multiple gestations. Surrogate parenting, although still not common, is another variation of planned parenthood that affects the mother-baby relationship.

The quest of the natural childbirth activists of the 1960s and 1970s to restore pregnancy and birth as normal nonmedical events, and breastfeeding as the expected way to feed the baby, has been gradually eclipsed by the expectation of parents that testing, monitoring, and measuring will ensure a healthier baby and mother.

Listening to Mothers Survey: A Snapshot of Birth and Breastfeeding in the United States

Juxtaposed against this rapidly changing picture of pregnancy and childbirth care is a relative resurgence in breastfeeding in the United States. It might be tempting to conclude, then, that increased medicalization of childbirth is not a problem for mothers planning to breastfeed. The Maternity Center Association's *Listening to Mothers* survey (LtM) is the first national survey that has asked women about their childbearing experiences, including postpartum care and breastfeeding.[1] It captures not only information about clinical care received, but also information on the attitudes, knowledge, and emotional perceptions about this care. A total of 1583 women who had babies in the United States between mid-2000 and mid-2002 were surveyed in May–June 2002, including a smaller number of eligible women identified through random digit telephone dialing and a majority who participated through an Internet panel. To develop a national profile of childbearing women, the data were adjusted with demographic and propensity score weightings using methodology developed and validated by Harris Interactive®.

The LtM survey findings show trends toward wide use of many interventions. These trends are troubling in light of previous chapters that have reviewed the direct and indirect influence that one or several of interventions combined may have on breastfeeding. Figure 12-1 summarizes key findings.

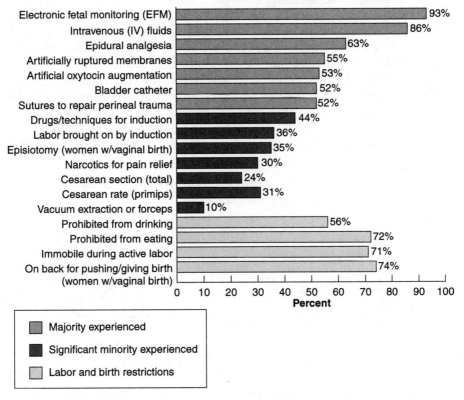

Labor and Birth Interventions

Intervention	Percent
Electronic fetal monitoring (EFM)	93%
Intravenous (IV) fluids	86%
Epidural analgesia	63%
Artificially ruptured membranes	55%
Artificial oxytocin augmentation	53%
Bladder catheter	52%
Sutures to repair perineal trauma	52%
Drugs/techniques for induction	44%
Labor brought on by induction	36%
Episiotomy (women w/vaginal birth)	35%
Narcotics for pain relief	30%
Cesarean section (total)	24%
Cesarean rate (primips)	31%
Vacuum extraction or forceps	10%
Prohibited from drinking	56%
Prohibited from eating	72%
Immobile during active labor	71%
On back for pushing/giving birth (women w/vaginal birth)	74%

Legend:
- Majority experienced
- Significant minority experienced
- Labor and birth restrictions

FIGURE 12-1 Labor and Birth Interventions and Restrictions: Selected Data from Listening to Mothers Survey. *Source: Declercq ER, Sakala C, Corry MP, et al. 2002. Listening to Mothers: Report of the First National U.S. Survey of Women's Childbearing Experiences.* New York: Maternity Center Association, October 2002. Used with permission of the Maternity Center Association and Harris Interactive.®

Given the evidence presented in previous chapters, the high prevalence of many of these interventions is of real concern. The 86% IV therapy rate, 35% episiotomy rate, and 93% EFM rate are inappropriately high, considering that 85% of all pregnancies are not expected to develop life-threatening conditions. The reported routine use of known non–evidence-based practices such as exclusive bed rest in labor (71%), withholding of food (72%) and oral fluids (56%), and supine position for delivery (74%), also suggests at best "culture lag" in the extreme and at worst a profound disregard for the evidence.

Cesarean Section and Vaginal Birth after Cesarean Trends

Previous chapters show that cesarean delivery, particularly unplanned cesarean, is associated with a cascade of interventions that impact breastfeeding. The LtM Survey findings on prevalence of cesarean sections mirror the nationally reported statistics, with a rate in 2001 of 24 % of total deliveries (see Chapter 8). This finding deserves additional discussion as the survey also found that a much higher percentage of cesarean births were in first-time mothers (31%). The United States cesarean section rate, persisting above 20% of all births since the mid-1980s, dropped for a short period in the mid-1990s, but has increased sharply since 1996 (Figure 12-2). Simultaneously, the vaginal birth after cesarean (VBAC) rate has

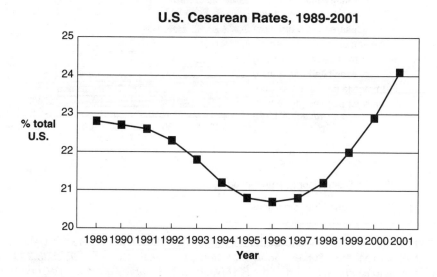

U.S. Cesarean Rates, 1989-2001

FIGURE 12-2 US Cesarean Rates, 1989–2001[6] *www.Cdc.gov/nchs. Pubs under Birth 2002. 1996 is the year of publication of the McMahan et al. study.*

decreased from a peak of 28.2% of eligible deliveries in 1998, to 20.7% in 2000 (the first year of the survey), to 16.4 % in 2001 (see Chapter 8, Figure 8-3). According to the survey discussion, "there was a strong annual trend in the data," with 25% of mothers who had previously given birth by cesarean and who gave birth 1–2 years before the survey being denied the option of a VBAC, while 58% of those with a previous cesarean who had given birth in the previous year were denied the option. As noted in Chapter 8, the reasons for this change come from a 1999 *Practice Bulletin* by the American College of Obstetricians and Gynecologists (ACOG) that emphasized the risks of VBAC, without explaining the risks of repeat cesarean section.[2] This bulletin sites one study as the evidence for this dramatic practice change.[3]

Goer has analyzed the considerable literature on safety of VBACs, including the McMahan et al. research cited by ACOG.[4] She concludes that VBAC is safer for the mother and equally safe for the baby, compared with repeat CS, when appropriate clinical criteria are met. In analyzing the McMahan et al. study, she questions their conclusions about VBAC having more "major complications" than repeat CS. Quoting from their findings that "major complications were nearly twice as likely among women undergoing trial of labor," Goer points out that Flamm identified another problem with this analysis:

> The authors coded wound infections and hemorrhage requiring transfusion as "minor complications." These would normally be considered major complications and coding them as such would have wiped out the difference [in risks between repeat CS and VBAC]. Even so, "nearly twice" the major complications rate amounted to a little less than 1 percent in the elective cesarean group, a little more than 1 percent in the VBAC group.[5]

This discussion on cesarean section and VBAC rates is intended to emphasize the point made in Chapter 2, which is that evidence can be interpreted differently by different individuals and also can be selectively ignored. Put another way, evidence can be in the eye of the beholder. *A Guide to Effective Care in Pregnancy and Childbirth*, based on Cochrane reviews when available and on other best available evidence when Cochrane reviews are not available, states the case clearly in a section entitled "Gap between evidence and practice":

> Obstetric practice has been slow to adopt the scientific evidence confirming the safety of vaginal birth after cesarean section. The degree of opposition to vaginal birth after cesarean section, in North America in particular, is difficult to explain, considering the strength of the evidence that vaginal birth after cesarean

is, under proper circumstances, both safe and effective. Two national consensus statements and two national professional bodies, in Canada and the United States, have policies of trial of labor after previous cesarean section. A randomized controlled trail of different strategies to encourage implementation of these policies showed that local opinion leaders were more effective than either national promulgation of guidelines or audit and feedback to obstetricians.[7]

The *Listening to Mothers* survey found that technology–intensive labor is the norm in the United States. This trend seems not to be a consumer-driven practice, according to survey findings. Mothers' attitudes about cesarean section showed that they preferred by 5 to 1 (83% compared to 16%) to try a vaginal birth when asked if for a future birth they had no medical reasons not to try vaginal birth and were offered elective cesarean. Mothers who recently had a vaginal birth were less likely to prefer a future cesarean (93% compared to 6%). The survey asked women if they agreed that "birth is a natural process that should not be interfered with unless absolutely medically necessary." A minority (19%) said they strongly agreed, and 26% said they somewhat agreed. Nearly one third of respondents, however, (31%) disagreed that birth is a natural process, and 24% had no opinion (Figure 12-3). This suggests that there may be a gradual erosion of the belief that childbirth is essentially natural, and is being replaced by the belief

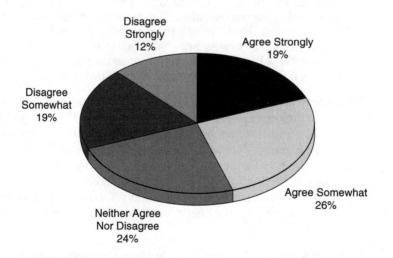

FIGURE 12-3 Responses to "Giving birth is a natural process that should not be interfered with unless medically necessary." *Source: Listening to Mothers Survey, 2002.* Used with permission of the Maternity Center Association and Harris Interactive.®

that it requires medical interference. A collaborator on the LtM survey emphasized that information was collected on many obstetrical interventions previously never studied on a national level and the findings point the way to additional studies. This survey is a descriptive snapshot of the experiences of women who gave birth in the U.S. from mid-2000 to mid-2002, and some aspects of obstetric care in this country, for example VBAC rates, are changing very quickly.[8]

Continuing with the "snapshot" of the current situation in the United States, the LtM survey findings on breastfeeding showed that 40% of women who delivered in hospitals had their babies in their arms in the first hour of birth, with 13% reporting their babies were in their partners' arms. However, 31% reported that their baby was with staff for "routine care" in the first hour and 14% were of babies were receiving "special care." At one week postpartum, 59% of respondents were exclusively breastfeeding. This is a drop from the 67% of total respondents who stated that as they neared the end of their pregnancy they had planned to exclusively breastfeed. Rooming-in is a known factor in promotion of early breastfeeding success. Findings from the LtM survey show that 45% of mothers who had cesarean section roomed-in with their babies, compared to 60% of vaginally delivered mothers. A significant finding was that 80% of mothers who planned exclusive breastfeeding received formula samples or offers from hospital personnel during postpartum hospital stay. There is no data on how many of these mothers delivered at a BFHI facility. However, the most current figure shows only 34 designated BFHI facilities, including 7 birth centers, 17 smaller and medium-sized hospitals, and 10 hospitals with level 3 nurseries that care for infants at risk.[9] The odds are small that mothers surveyed delivered in a 'Baby-Friendly' hospital.

Birthing and Breastfeeding: Still Separate in the Literature

Recently published is a comprehensive book on breastfeeding, *Reclaiming Breastfeeding for the United States*.[10] The book analyzes breastfeeding from many perspectives and reviews breastfeeding policy and practice environment in light of both international and national trends. It gives an update on the Baby Friendly Hospital Initiative in the United States and explores its successes and limitations. What is disappointing about the book is that it fails to analyze breastfeeding outcomes against the backdrop of obstetrical practices. In over 200 pages of text, only one page addresses childbirth anesthesia as a possible negative factor in breastfeeding outcomes.

Dennis conducted an extensive review of literature published in the decade 1990–2000 on breastfeeding initiation and duration to delineate effective strategies for positive change in the North American setting.[11] The author's discussion on interventions that affect breastfeeding includes a short section on intrapartum experience, and she cites the Riordan study discussed in Chapter 6. While acknowledging that the study shows that labor medicines negatively influence early feeding, she mentions that this study showed no long-term differences in breastfeeding duration at 6 weeks. Dennis fails to look at the bigger picture. The observers in the Riordan study were all certified lactation consultants and this fact could account for the long-term findings. The services of lactation specialists are among the reasons breastfeeding rates are not lower, as they are helping to "fix" the problems created in childbirth.

The fact that many U.S. hospitals now have lactation consultants on staff is a positive development. Twenty-five years ago breastfeeding mothers had to rely on their pediatric care providers, family members, local La Leche League, or simply muddle through difficulties themselves. However, the presence of lactation consultants may be a confounding factor in evaluating breastfeeding outcomes because their intensive assistance to mothers with problems may enable breastfeeding success in the long run. In the words of Ruth Wester, a breastfeeding specialist who has worked with mothers and babies and breastfeeding for over 30 years, "Why do so many of these babies who should be doing fine, present with oral motor behaviors detrimental to breastfeeding success, bonding, and attachment? We can no longer ignore probable impact of current birthing practices on these issues. Our babies deserve a better beginning."[12]

Global Trends in Pregnancy, Childbirth, and Breastfeeding

This picture of pregnancy care in the United States is in marked contrast to that in developing countries. Persistently high maternal mortality rates claim the lives of nearly 600,000 women annually. Infant mortality rates, while dropping, are still high. In these

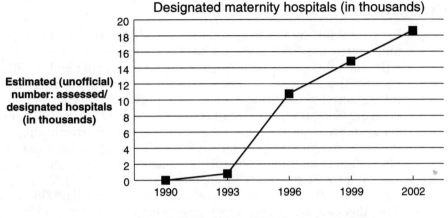

Source: UNICEF New York from UNICEF Country Programs Reports.

FIGURE 12-4   Global Trends in Baby-friendly Hospitals.

settings priorities are different. A "safe" birth seems more important than a "good" or mother-friendly birth. Yet, as pointed out in
Chapter 1, there should not a distinction—a "safe" birth is one in
which the mother feels safe and cared for. Breastfeeding has been
included in Safe Motherhood programs, but the links are weak
and the benefits of breastfeeding for the mother herself are often
not appreciated.

In resource-poor countries, breastfeeding in the early months
continues to mean life or death to the infant. The chance of dying
at two months of age or less is five times higher if the infant does
not breastfeed. This relative risk remains high throughout the first
year of life.[13]

The global Baby Friendly Hospital Initiative has grown in
the decade since it was launched. At the end of 2002, more than
18,000 maternity hospitals had been designated as BFHI globally.[14] The Innocenti Declaration was signed August 1, 1990,
identifying the practice of the Ten Steps in all maternity services as an operational target. BFHI was developed in 1991,
piloted in 12 countries, and inaugurated as a global initiative
in 1992. In the ensuing 10 years, breastfeeding has been promoted through the BFHI in 135 countries, and 79 countries
have initiated activities to establish codes of marketing breast
milk substitutes. (See Figure 12-4.)

HIV/AIDS, Birth, and Breastfeeding

Progress made by the International Code of Marketing Breastmilk Substitutes and BFHI activities has been overshadowed in Africa, Asia, and other parts of the world where the impact of the HIV/AIDS pandemic on maternity care has been profound. Maternal and infant mortality are rising in many countries and gains in child survival are being reversed.[15] Mother-to-child transmission of HIV can occur in pregnancy, childbirth, and as a result of breastfeeding.[16] Pregnant mothers in hard-hit areas, far from expecting a routine ultrasound or multiple laboratory tests, need essential prenatal care. They may wait for hours in crowded, understaffed facilities that may lack basic medicines to treat anemia and malaria. Midwives and other care providers do their best under often the most difficult of circumstances. Planning for delivery and deciding about the safest infant feeding becomes a complex issue if a mother has tested HIV positive. International guidelines for HIV-infected mothers have remained clear that mothers need counseling to make an informed choice about how to feed. The global recommendation is that exclusive breastfeeding is still best for mothers who are HIV negative or of unknown status (see Box 12-1).

Box 12-1   Infant Feeding Guidelines for HIV-Infected Mothers, 1997 and 2000

- "The risk of replacement feeding should be less than the potential risk of HIV transmission through infected breastmilk so that infant illness and death do not increase. Otherwise, there is no advantage in replacement feeding."[17]
- "For mothers who are HIV negative or who do not know their HIV status: exclusive breastfeeding for the first 6 months and continued breastfeeding for up to 2 years or longer with the addition of complementary food after 6 months is recommended. If, however, a woman has tested positive for HIV, and when replacement feeding is acceptable, feasible, affordable, sustainable, and safe, avoidance of all breastfeeding by HIV-positive mothers is recommended. Otherwise, exclusive breastfeeding is recommended during the first months of life."[18]

The issue of HIV transmission in childbirth care in resource-poor settings has not received as much attention as infant feeding counseling, in spite of the fact that this is one of the most likely times that HIV can be vertically transmitted.[16] Funding and programming have focused on treatment during labor with anti-retroviral medicines and underplayed the importance of safe labor and delivery management. Keeping labor and birth normal can reduce risks of HIV transmission to the fetus. Ironically, the practices of routine rupture of membranes to speed labor, routine cutting of episiotomy, forceps and vacuum delivery, and the vigorous suctioning of the newborn *are all discouraged because of the risks of HIV transmission.*[19] For HIV-positive mothers who have chosen to breastfeed, exclusive breastfeeding is more important than ever, because the biggest danger is from mixed feeding.[20] Homebirth care providers must know the basic facts about mother-to-child transmission and must be empowered to protect themselves and their mothers and babies as much as possible. They can also provide important feeding support in the postpartum period (see Figure 12-5).

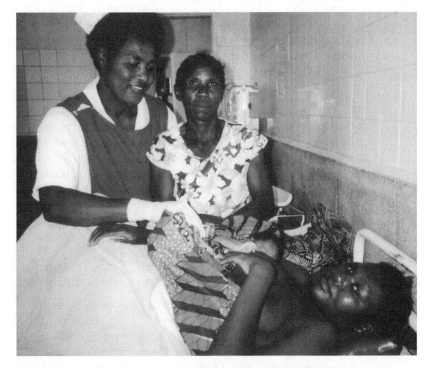

FIGURE 12-5   In Ndola, Zambia, where the HIV prevalence in pregnancy reaches up to 40%, delivery care includes no routine episiotomy, no routine suctioning, and skin-to-skin contact and initiation of breastfeeding. This mother does not know her HIV status.[21] *Photo by Mary Kroeger, 2000.*

Challenges Ahead: Advocacy and Activism

A socio-anthropological perspective presented in "The Resurgence of Breastfeeding at the End of the Second Millennium" paints in broad brushstrokes the history, major clinical practice, and behavior changes in breastfeeding over the last century.[22] These authors analyze the evidence for why, after gradual decline, there has again been an increase in breastfeeding in North America in the last 20 years of the twentieth century. In their summary section they write:

> There is no evidence that health-care providers are providing more support for breastfeeding, and most of the international and national policies postdated the resurgence of breastfeeding, although they may have influenced the upswing in the 1990s. A more plausible explanation of the resurgence in breastfeeding in all segments of society is the pervasive influence of the natural childbirth movement of the 1960s and 1970s, with its effects on the standard management of childbirth. In addition, the increase of breastfeeding among low income women may be attributable in part to programmatic changes in the provision of supplemental food through the WIC program (Chapter 1) and targeting of breastfeeding promotion efforts to the specific concerns of these women.

Their conclusions corroborate the thesis of this book, that childbirth and breastfeeding are by nature interrelated. Although breastfeeding rates are increasing in the United States from past decades, they point out that by no means have rates increased so as to meet national goals. They suggest that "the strategies likely to have a lasting effect on future breastfeeding rates will be societal pressures that affect existing breastfeeding barriers."

National-Level Advocacy

We have come full circle back to the need for a movement for both mother- and baby-friendly care. Fortunately, several such movements already exist and are growing in strength. These include:

- *Coalition to Improve Maternity Services (CIMS) in the USA:* CIMS has already merged the BFHI assessment process with a broader-scoped assessment of mother friendly care. The CIMS Ten Steps to a Mother Friendly Childbirth Initiative include BFHI's Ten Steps to Successful Breastfeeding as the MFCI tenth step.

- *Better Birth Initiative in South Africa:* Better Births Initiative has piloted MF care in multiracial South Africas and the initiative springs from a platform of evidence-based care. Part of their initiative is to provide electronic copies of the WHO Reproductive Health Library, a wealth of information and teaching tools, with the evidence that supports a model of low-intervention childbirth.

- *Relacahupan:* The movement for "humanizing of childbirth" has 20 member countries in South America, Central America, and the Caribbean, and each of these countries has a national organization. Organized after the second Fortaleza Brazil meeting in 2001, a main goal of the movement is the reversal of the cesarean section rates in member countries.

- *Childbirth and Breastfeeding Foundation of Thailand (CBFT):* Founded in 1998, this Thai group has developed a mother- and baby-friendly model of maternity care. They also strongly advocate for mothers and young children through a daughter organization, BAMBI.

More information on these organizations, including Web site addresses, can be found in the Appendices.

Global Advocacy

- *WHO/European Regional Office, Perinatal Task Force, the Perinatal Course, and the Bologna Score:* In January 2000, the WHO European Regional Office convened a meeting in which participants developed key indicators for the evaluation of effective care of normal labor.[22] Task Force concerns were that labor was being considered as "abnormal" in increasingly and unjustifiably large proportions in many countries, consuming scare resources that could be much better directed toward genuinely abnormal pregnancies and labors. The key indicator was made up of five measures of effective management of normal childbirth and early breastfeeding, and was named the "Bologna Score," after the venue of the meeting. Two additional indicators were "qualifiers" to assist with understanding the overall environment of labor management.

- *World Alliance of Breastfeeding Action (WABA):* WABA was founded on February 14, 1991 and is a global network of organizations and individuals who believe breastfeeding is the right of all children and mothers and who dedicate themselves to protect, promote, and support this right. WABA acts on the Innocenti Declaration and works in liaison with UNICEF. WABA has embraced mother-friendly and humane childbirth as an adjunct to breastfeeding promotion. The WABA World Breastfeeding Week Action Folder is issued annually prior to World Breastfeeding Week in August. The 2002 WBW Action Folder contained advocacy information on humane and natural childbirth and included a shortened version of the CIMS Mother Friendly Childbirth Ten Steps as an example. In April 2002, WABA launched the Global Initiative for Mother Support (GIMS), a mother-support oriented initative that also includes empowered and human childbirth in its platform. In September 2002, the second WABA Global Forum was held in Arusha, Tanzania. A series of workshops on birthing practices brought together researchers and advocates for linking childbirth and breastfeeding (Figure 12-6). As a result of this forum WABA has committed to strengthening the dialogue with WHO and UNICEF about broadening BFHI to include childbirth practices.

Challenges in Professional Education: Thinking Outside the Box

It was recognized in the late 1980s, as the Ten Steps of BFHI where being formulated, that more than half of all babies in the world are not born in maternity facilities. However, it was also recognized that maternity facilities are where the obstetric and pediatric standards and policies are developed and implemented. Thus, the WHO/UNICEF Joint Statement targeted maternity hospitals. The BFHI assessment criteria ask if all staff members that care for mothers and babies are trained in the implementation of appropriate breastfeeding policy. This question must now be extended to the rest of maternity care: labor and birth.

Obstetrical care providers must be able to mentally put themselves in the place of a newborn: imagining the grogginess and disorientation of medications, the pain of early procedures, and the anguish at early separation from a mother who might be recovering from a long, difficult delivery. Pediatric care providers need to imagine themselves flat on their backs, legs in stirrups, with tubes and wires and blinking machines attached to them. In

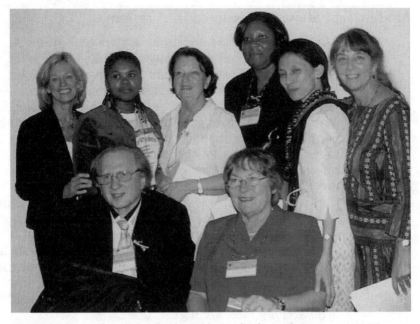

FIGURE 12-6 Global childbirth and breastfeeding advocates at WABA Global Forum 2002 in Tanzania. Clockwise from top left: Rae Davies (USA, doula and exec. director CIMS), Ntombaza Makinana (South Africa, midwife, BBI), Anna-Berit Ransjo-Arvidson (Sweden, midwife-researcher), Maureen Chilila (Zambia, midwife, Woman Friendly Services Project), Mel Habanananda (Thailand, midwife, founder CBFT), Mary Kroeger (USA, midwife and author), Ann-Marie Widstrom (Sweden, midwife-researcher), Dr. Adik Levin, (Estonia, neonatologist, Human Neonatal Care Initiative). *Photo by WABA Staff.*

a resource-poor setting, they need to imagine themselves as young mothers referred by the village midwife for a complication, lying on a hard bed, with no family nearby, not knowing what frightening procedures are planned and terrified that they may die. This is the kind of reorientation that is needed to allow for holistic maternity care.

Childbirth educators and doulas must put themselves in the shoes of the lactation counselors and specialists. All involved in childbirth and newborn care need to know the basics of how to keep labor normal and on track, how to keep mother and baby together, and how to assist with breastfeeding.

Models That Show Professional Integration

- *Midwifery Model of Care:* Midwives are trained to be experts in normal birth and are usually also skilled at assisting with breastfeeding. However, training midwives in refresher courses in many countries has shown that nurses and midwives often lack knowledge and skills on how to keep birth normal and how to support mothers in labor in a caring way. For breastfeeding support, they may know the correct "messages" but do not know how to ensure that breastfeeding gets off to the right start. Increasingly, midwifery practice in the industrialized countries is being more medicalized. In the United States, more and more nurse-midwives are trained to assist at cesarean delivery, to perform vacuum extraction, and to assist in provision of epidural anesthesic, but lack practice in low-technology care for normal childbirth. Midwifery and perinatal nursing education must include experience in birth centers and/or homebirth, where childbirth is allowed to progress without medical interventions and where breastfeeding rates are high.

- *Wellstart International Lactation Management Education Program:* Multisectoral teams may be effective, as shown by the model promoted by Wellstart International (WSI). Between 1983 and 1998, WSI, located in San Diego, California, offered a four-week entry-level postgraduate training course in lactation management education (LME) for health professionals from developing countries. Their strategy was to encourage participation in multidisciplinary country teams made up, ideally, of an obstetrician, a pediatrician, a senior nurse or midwife, a nutritionist, and a public health administrator or government representative. The goal with this LME program was to "contribute to the sustained promotion, protection, and support of breastfeeding (including maternal nutrition, complementary feeding, and the contraceptive effects of exclusive breastfeeding) in developing nations as a means of improving infant and maternal health."[24] Spanning 15 years, the Wellstart International LME program trained 653 participants from 55 countries, and the course was offered in English, Spanish, French, and Russian. Wellstart's program also included follow-up support and continuing education back at the national levels. Many of the global leaders in BFHI and change agents in national and regional public health programs attended this course. A model similar to this approach, which includes additional training on intrapartum care, is needed if we are to have mother- and baby-friendly maternity care.

- *The WHO Essential Antenatal, Perinatal, and Postpartum Care Course:* The WHO Regional Office for Europe has developed an Antenatal, Perinatal, and Postpartum Care Course for maternity care providers.[25] This course, made up of 28 modules, can be taught in short sessions or in one longer course lasting five to six days. *A Guide to Effective Care in Pregnancy and Childbirth* serves as the foundation text, and trainers are prepared to be familiar with all of the modular content and the teaching materials. Not only is the course comprehensive—spanning pregnancy, intrapartum, and postpartum care—but it also strives to promote the Perinatal Principles endorsed by the WHO-Euro Perinatal Task Force. These include:
  - Care for normal labor and birth should be demedicalized.
  - Care should be based on the use of appropriate technology.
  - Care should be evidence based.
  - Care should be regionalized and based on an efficient system of referral.
  - Care should be multidisciplinary.
  - Care should be holistic.
  - Care should be family centered.
  - Care should be culturally appropriate.
  - Care should involved women in the decision making.
  - Care should respect the privacy, dignity, and confidentiality of women.

The course has been offered since 1999 and has been taught in Kazakhstan, Turkmenistan, Kyrgystan, Uzbekistan, Tajikistan, Belarus, Moldova, Kosovo, Georgia, Armenia, and Russia. Most of these countries had been isolated during Soviet rule from updated research in perinatal care and practiced in a rigid, highly medicalized and non-mother- and baby-friendly manner. The course continues to be offered and is an excellent way to begin to sensitize staff to the need to change. Clinical practice is a very small part of the course, and more extensive training and mentoring are necessary to really change outdated, non-evidence-based practices.[24] Three months after training, a follow-up visit is made by trainers to evaluate progress in implementing change and adopting the new approaches.

Challenges in Research Agendas: Breaking Through the Cul-de-Sac

The research by Righard and Alade on inborn breastfeeding seeking behavior has been much quoted in this book, and is well known among breastfeeding advocates for its presentation of previously undescribed inborn newborn feeding behaviors that are significantly disturbed by separating the newborn from the mother for bathing and weighing.[26] These were the sentinel findings on which Step Four of BFHI was based. Findings in this study of equally high significance were that pethidine (Demerol) given to the mother in labor disturbs this same early feeding behavior, but these results have not received the same attention in breastfeeding promotion and practice. This omission is unfortunate since multiple research studies have confirmed that maternal medication with pethidine is linked to neonatal respiratory depression, early disturbances in breastfeeding, and other newborn behaviors (see Chapter 6). Mothers need to be informed about this and breastfeeding advocates need to stop the use of pethidine.

Niles Newton called this persistent retaining of outdated, even harmful, practices and not acting on new research evidence "culture lag." Michel Odent calls it "circular" versus "cul-de-sac" epidemiology when researchers selectively look at some research issues repeatedly while selectively ignoring others. Henci Goer makes a stronger case against "spin doctoring the evidence," misrepresenting the research in order to serve professional, personal, or economic agendas. There must be more unbiased research that looks at childbirth management, birth outcomes, and breastfeeding as a continuum. As Linda Smith puts it, we must begin to "connect the dots."

Restoring the Continuum

Health care providers, childbirth educators, doulas, breastfeeding care providers and parents must embrace and act on the evidence. In a truly normal childbirth process, both mother and newborn are hormonally "programmed" with beta-endorphins, catacholamines, physiologic levels of oxytocin, along with other factots still not well understood. Optimally with attentive, noninterventive support the dyad will transition through the safe delivery of the placenta, through the change from fetal to newborn circula-

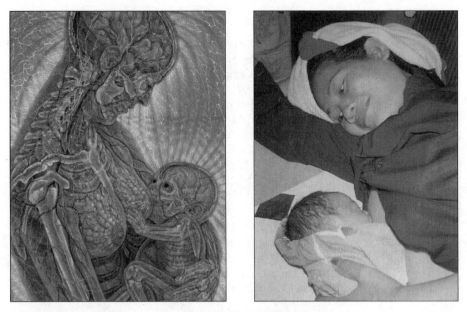

FIGURES 12-7 AND 12-8   Nature's plan: The mother-baby continuum.
Left—*Nursing* by Alex Gray
Right—Cambodian mother and newborn. *Photo by Mary Kroeger.*

tion, through the first breath of extrauterine life. When the baby
lies skin-to-skin with the mother, covered and warm, they move
to the first moments of touching, cuddling, and bonding without
any major interventions by care providers. Left undisturbed and
safe, mother and baby will continue this transition to breastfeeding, each helping and adjusting to the other, guided by ancient
instinct and responding to rushes of hormones. Thus the continuum is intact.

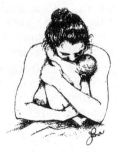

References

1. Declercq ER, Sakala C, Corry MP, Applebaum S, Risher P. 2002. *Listening to Mothers: Report of the First National U.S. Survey of Women's Childbearing Experiences.* New York: Maternity Center Association, October 2002.

2. American College of Obstetricians and Gynecologists. 1999. *ACOG Practice Bulletin #5, Vaginal Birth after Previous Cesarean Section.* American College of Obstetricians and Gynecologists, Washington, DC.

3. McMahan MJ, Luther ER, Bowes WA, Olshan AF. 1996. Comparison of a trial of labor with an elective second cesarean section. *N Engl J Med,* 335:689–695.

4. Goer H. 2003. A consumer viewpoint: Spin-doctoring the research. *Birth* 30(2):124–129.

5. Flamm BL. 1997. Once a cesarean, always a controversy. *Obstet Gynecol,* 90:312–315.

6. Data for graph from NCHS Hospital Discharge Surveys. *www.cdc.gov/nchs.* Pubs under Birth 2002 US Cesarean Rates, 1989–2001.

7. Enkin M, Keirse M, Renfrew M, et al. 2000. *A Guide to Effective Care in Pregnancy and Childbirth,* 3rd ed. Oxford: Oxford University Press.

8. Sakala Carol. 2003. Personal communication.

9. Cadwell Karin. 2003. Personal communication.

10. Cadwell K (Ed.). 2002. *Reclaiming Breastfeeding for the United States.* Boston: Jones and Bartlett Publishers.

11. Dennis C. 2002. Breastfeeding initiation and duration: A 1990-2000 literature review. *JOGNN,* 31(1):12–32.

12. Wester R. 2003. Lactation specialist, Wellstart International. Personal communication.

13. WHO. 2000. WHO Collaborative Study Team on the Role of Breastfeeding on the Prevention of Infant Mortality—Effect of breastfeeding on infant and child mortality due to infections disease in less developed countries: A pooled analysis. *Lancet,* 355(9202):451–455.

14. UNICEF. 2003. UNICEF Report on Progress on the WHO/UNICEF Baby-Friendly Hospital Initiative (BFHI), presented by Miriam Labbok at the "WHO Consultancy on the Global Strategy on Infant and Young Child Feeding," February 10, 2003.

15. Israel E, Kroeger M. 2003. Integrating Prevention of Mother-to-child HIV Transmission into Existing Maternal, Child, and Reproductive Health Programs. *Technical Guidance Series,* No 3. January 2003. Boston: Pathfinder International. *www.pathfind.org.*

16. DeCock KM, Fowler E, Mercier E, et al. 2000. Prevention of mother-to-child HIV transmission in resource poor countries. *JAMA,* 23(9):175–182.
17. UNAIDS, WHO, UNICEF. 1997. *HIV and Infant Feeding.* A policy statement developed collaboratively by UNAIDS, WHO, UNICEF. Geneva.
18. WHO. 2000. New data on the prevention of mother-to-child transmission of HIV and their policy implications: Conclusions and recommendations. WHO Technical Consultation on Behalf of the UNFPA/UNICEF/WHO/UNAIDS Interagency Task Force Team on Mother-to-Child transmission of HIV, Geneva, 11–13 October 2000.
19. WHO. 1999. *HIV in Pregnancy: A Review.* Geneva: WHO/CHS/RHR/99.15
20. Coutsoudis A, Pillay K, Kuhn L, et al. 2001. Method of feeding and transmission of HIV-1 from mothers-to-children by 15 months of age: Prospective cohort study. South Africa, Vitamin A Study Group. *AIDS,* 15(3):379–387.
21. Ntombela N, Kroeger M. 2001. Ndola Demonstration Project: Midwives take the lead to reduce mother-to-child transmission of HIV. *Quickening,* No. 3. May/June. 15–17.
22. Wright A, Schandler R. 2001. The Resurgence of Breastfeeding at the End of the Second Millennium. *J Nutr,* 131(2):421S–5S.
23. Chalmers B, Porter R. 2001. Assessing effective care in normal labor: The Bologna Score. *Birth,* 28(2):79–83.
24. Wellstart International. 1998. The Lactation Management Education Experience 1983–1998. Accomplishments, lessons learned, and recommended strategies. Submitted as the final report to the Office of Health and Nutrition, United States Agency for International development. March 31, 1998.
25. Chalmers B. 2003. Personal communication.
26. Righard L, Alade MO. 1990. Effect of delivery room routines on success of first breast-feed. *Lancet,* 336:1105–1107.

THE COALITION FOR IMPROVING MATERNITY SERVICES (CIMS)

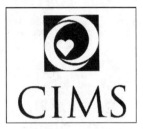

CIMS was established in 1996 as a collaborative effort among a broad spectrum of maternity service providers, including midwives, physicians, nurses, childbirth educators, labor support and postpartum doulas, and lactation consultants. The extraordinary founding meeting called together childbirth and breastfeeding activists, including Marshall Klaus, Ina May Gaskin, and Suzanne Arms, to name a few. In its first five years, the work of CIMS has focused on the creation and implementation of the evidence-based *Mother-Friendly Childbirth Initiative (MFCI)*, which provides guidelines for identifying and designating "mother-friendly" birth sites including hospitals, birth centers, and home-birth services. The initiative outlines ten steps for mother-friendly care and includes a requirement for birth sites to also qualify as "baby-friendly" according to the World Health Organization's guidelines. A consumer version of the Initiative, *"Having a Baby? Ten Questions to Ask"* is also available in English, Spanish, French, and Czech.

In 2001 and 2002, the MF Assessment tools and process were piloted and two facilities in the United States—Northern New Mexico Women's Health Center in Taos, NM and Three Rivers were assessed. In Feb 2002, both were designated as MF Facilities. Some controversy has ensued since then as the Taos birth center has not proceeded to gain the full BFHI designation. The founding members have agreed that full MF designation requires Baby-Friendly USA designation. Additional facilities are awaiting assessment and this exciting movement, within the process. The CIMS Website is *www.motherfriendly.org*

THE BETTER BIRTHS INITIATIVE (BBI)

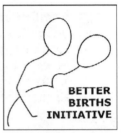

BBI was developed by health professionals in South Africa in 2000 with international participation to help provide a better quality of childbirth care for women and improve maternal outcomes in low-income countries where resources are limited and better services will reduce maternal mortality. It is a focused set of standards that are evidence based and aim to improve the quality and humanity of obstetric care at delivery using existing resources. The initiative targets health care providers and assists them in understanding research evidence, making decisions about best practices, and establishing implementation procedures to assure change. It encourages health workers to abandon practices that are painful, potentially harmful, and have no evidence of benefit.

BBI is a project that started in Coronation Hospital in South Africa in the Effective Care Research Unit. It is a component of the *Effective Health Care Alliance Programme* (EHCAP), supported by the Department for International Development. Funds for South Africa activities come from a variety of sources, including the Government of South Africa.

Project Objective—The objective of this pilot study is to test the effectiveness of an educational package, which focuses on a few key areas of midwifery and obstetric care, to bring about change in obstetric practice.

Preliminary results—Exit interviews show that use of enemas has been reduced at nine sites, and episiotomy and shaving were used less at follow-up at seven sites (comparison by study group is ongoing). Labour ward staff found other procedures (companionship, non-supine position) more difficult to change with existing facilities and resources. Three out of five intervention sites used the self-audit, and feedback during in-depth interviews suggested it stimulated discussion around change and motivated staff.

Interactive Workshop—Change in practice is possible using a 2-hour interactive workshop. The educational package is being modified, in light of the study findings, for use in other provinces in South Africa. A low-tech, low-cost version is being piloted in Eastern Cape. There is interest internationally (China, Pakistan, Nigeria) to adapt and implement the package. Selected materials are available in the WHO Reproductive Health Library (2001), and all materials will be available in downloadable format from the website: *www.liv.ac.uk/lstm/ehcap/bbimainpage*

WHO Reproductive Health Library (RHL)

The WHO RHL is promoted by the BBI. The WHO Reproductive Health Library is "An affordable, accessible, and user-friendly source of up-to-date evidence for reproductive health care in developing countries."

The WHO Reproductive Health Library (RHL) is an annual electronic review journal that focuses on evidence-based solutions to reproductive health problems in low and middle-income countries. The RHL contains systematic reviews on reproductive health topics, expert commentaries on the relevance of the findings, and practical aspects with management recommendations. A new feature in RHL is 'implementation aids;' these are materials designed to help health professionals use research evidence in practice. Selected Better Births Initiative materials are available on RHL 5 (2002).

Subscription to the RHL (CD-ROM) is free to individuals in low and middle-income countries. To subscribe, send your postal details to: WHO Reproductive Health Library, Special Programme of Research, Development and Research Training in Human Reproduction, World Health Organization, CH-1211 Geneva 27, Switzerland. Tel: +41 22 791 3380; Fax: +41 22 791 4171; Email: RHL@who.int

APPENDIX C

RELACAHUPAN (THE LATIN AMERICAN AND CARIBBEAN NETWORK FOR THE HUMANIZATION OF THE CHILDBIRTH)

(Adapted from the Spanish)

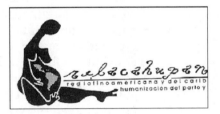

RELACAHUPAN is a set of national networks, groupings and people who propose to improve the experience of the childbirth and the form to be born. They first came together at the Congress "Humanización of the Childbirth and the Birth" in Ceará, Brazil, in November of 2000. As of that date more people of diverse countries who had not been able to attend that congress have joined.

The groups or people of each country have action autonomy, but we are united in the work to improve the life in the planet by means of a healthy and satisfactory childbirth and a birth. By means of the Network, the groups and people interchange information and interact like part of a continental campaign by the humanización of the childbirth.

There is also the aim to reduce the high Cesarean section rates in urban Latin America and de-medicalized childbirth in general. In Chile, Columbia and Mexico the many private facilities have

over 50% CS (Belizan, 1999). Argentine, Brazil, Paraguay have
40% National CS rates.

Objectives [Author's note: these are taken from the Spanish translation to the English on the website]

- To promote the humanización, and thus the
  redescubrimiento of which it is normal during the reproductive and neonatal cycle.
- To favor, from before the pregnancy, the rights and the pro-
  tagónico role of the woman and the baby who is born, offering a secure atmosphere to them, confidence and respect, in
  addition to ensure technical abilities of those who we will
  accompany them in this stage.
- To recognize the potential of the partera professional and
  traditional (Professional and Traditional midwife) in the
  gaining of this goal, attention to its necessities and realities
  and in special consideration that they attend populations
  which are marginalized.
- To cause the conducive beginning and evolution of strategies and actions to the improvement of programs and gov-
  ernmental policies with base in scientific evidences.
- To spread information and to carry out studies on models
  and beneficial practices in the attention to the childbirth, as
  much in modern systems as in indigenous systems.
- To incorporate the recommendations on the safe attention to
  the propose childbirth by the WHO.

Relacahupan Member Countries:

- *Americas of the South:* Argentine, Bolivia, Brazil, Childe,
  Columbia, Ecuador, Peru, Uruguay, Venezuela.
- *Meso America:* Costa Rica, El Salvador, Mexico, Nicaragua.
- *Caribbean:* Bahamas, Jamaica, Puerto Rico, Dominican
  Republic, St Thomas, Trinidad, and Tobago.

Contact Information:

Meso America: *mesoamerica@relacahupan.org*
Caribbean: *caribe@relacahupan.org*
Americas of the South: *delsur@relacahupan.org*

CHILDBIRTH & BREASTFEEDING FOUNDATION OF THAILAND (CBFT)

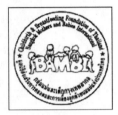

Formed in 1998 in recognition of the need to decrease use of expensive birth technology, to stop the rising cesarean section rate, and to bring about greater awareness of the value of natural childbirth and breastfeeding.

Mission statement

CBFT is a non-profit networking and resource centre based in Bangkok, Thailand, dedicated to ensuring the best possible start in life for our babies. We believe that this can best be achieved through:

- Encouraging the appropriate use of technology and medication for all births.
- Promoting breastfeeding for every mother and baby in the community.
- Providing information and training to health professionals involved in maternity care.
- Supporting parents through the pregnancy, birth and post-natal period.

Contacts: For more information about CBFT contact:

English Speaking: Mel Habanananda email: *meltanit@asiaac-cess.net.th* or Meena Sobsamai email: *sobsamai@cscoms.com*

Thai speaking: Ton email: *ton@box1.a-net.net.th*

BAMBI (Bangkok Babies & Mothers International) is a project of the *Childbirth & Breastfeeding Foundation of Thailand* (CBFT). BAMBI was formed in 1982 when a small group of women who had been attending prenatal classes together in Bangkok decided to continue meeting once a month after their babies were born. Their general aim was to give the mothers of babies and young children support and friendship, and to help them with any problems that might arise from the sense of loneliness and isolation that sometimes comes from living in a large city such as Bangkok.

AIMS AND OBJECTIVES: BAMBI is a mother-led, non-profit group, offering support and companionship in the early years of parenthood. We hold monthly and weekly playgroups for babies and toddlers, organise Christmas parties, Bring & Buy Sales, Summer playgroup, and Splash parties, to mention a few. Our charities section is very active, with a focus on helping other children in Bangkok. We also meet twice a month for discussions on breastfeeding and natural birth, support for which is difficult to come by in Bangkok. *www.bambi-bangkok.org/CBFT/CBFT.htm*

THE WORLD ALLIANCE FOR BREASTFEEDING ACTION (WABA)

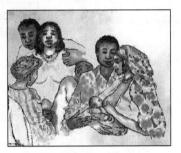

The World Alliance for Breastfeeding Action was formed on February 14, 1991. WABA is a global network of organizations and individuals who believe breastfeeding is the right of all children and mothers and who dedicate themselves to protect, promote, and support this right. WABA acts on the Innocenti Declaration and works in liaison with UNICEF.

WABA's goals:

- Re-establish and maintain a global breastfeeding culture
- Eliminate all obstacles to breastfeeding
- Promote more regional and national level cooperation
- Advocate for breastfeeding in development, women, and environmental programmes

WABA's Role

Information sharing and networking:

- To strengthen and coordinate existing activities to create more momentum
- To build bridges among all breastfeeding advocates: grass roots groups and individuals, UN agencies, governments, and international NGOs
- Stimulate and support new and collaborative efforts

Alliance Building: WABA recognizes the importance of national breastfeeding alliances and alliances among all supporters of breastfeeding. The initiator of a national network affiliated to WABA should be committed to an open and inclusive process involving all individuals and organizations that protect, promote, and support breastfeeding.

WABA activities involving birthing practices:

- WBW Action Folder 2002—addresses birthing and breast-feeding
- WABA Global Forum II 2002—Birthing Practices as a Core Workshop Theme
- Health Care Practices Task Force

WABA website: *www.waba.org.my/*

Global Initiative on Mother Support (GIMS)

GIMS, launched in April 2002, is a global initiative coordinated by the Mother Support Task Force of the World Alliance for Breast-feeding Action (WABA), and aims to create the appropriate environment of awareness and support for a mother to initiate and sustain breastfeeding. As defined by GIMS, mother support is any support provided to mothers for the purpose of improving breastfeeding practices for both mother and baby. The support needed varies from woman to woman but generally includes encouragement, accurate and timely information, humane care during childbirth, advice, reassurance, affirmation, hands-on assistance, and practical tips.

GIMS goals:

- To broaden the support for mothers beyond the breastfeeding period, to include support during pregnancy, birth and post-natal
- To develop guidelines and tools for transforming birthing practices that specifically affect breastfeeding into a more humane and gender sensitive health care practice
- To promote a global understanding of mother support that values, gives credibility, and strengthens community-based mother support programmes and networks
- To promote Step 10 of the BFHI, and develop guidelines for putting it into effect by broadening the understanding of breastfeeding support groups

- To link and collaborate with other issue movements such as those working on natural/humane childbirth practices, family support, midwifery, women's health and rights, etc. in order to facilitate a holistic view on mother support
- To provide the impetus for changes in employment, health facility, and marketplace policies and practices so that women experience optimal pregnancy, birthing, and breast-feeding outcomes.

ZAMBIA: LUSAKA WOMAN-FRIENDLY SERVICES PROJECT

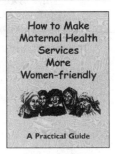

Zambia, a southern African country with one of the highest maternal mortality rates in the world at 649/100,000 (Zambia DHS, 1996) has been trying to improve quality of the maternal and neonatal care in order to address this critical situation. There are reports that maternity hospital care is not women-centered, nor does it provides care that reinforces keeping birth as normal as possible. A prospective observational study was conducted in 1994-95 of 84 Zambian obstetrically normal mothers who were admitted and delivered in eleven maternity facilities (Maimbolwa, et al. 1997).

Findings showed that the majority of women were confined to bed during the entire labor and delivery, food and drink was withheld, no gowns were provided, and none were allowed a companion in labor. In addition, fetal monitoring was inadequate and the partograph (tool for monitoring labor progress) was inconsistently used. At delivery, all women were placed in the lithotomy position, primiparas were strapped in stirrups, and there was a general lack of support for early mother-baby contact, for prevention of hypothermia, or for early initiation of breastfeeding. It is worth noting that there has been an active Baby Friendly Hospital Initiative in Zambia since 1992, but recent budget constraints have prevented the both the expansion of BFHI and the reassessment of existing BF hospitals.

Recently the General Nursing Council in Zambia has revised the nursing and midwifery curriculum introducing "evidence based practices" in the training school and clinical sites (abstract #IH 38486 APHA Meeting 2002). New practices have included companionship in labor, restriction of routine episiotomy, and allowing the mother to choose her position for labor and delivery. A short user-friendly guide for health service mangers has been developed by the Lusaka Woman-friendly Services Project (International Perinatal Care Unit, ICH, UK, 2000). This booklet, *How to Make Maternal Health Services More Woman-friendly*, provides low cost tools for improving the quality of services in reproductive health. It starts from the premise that both technical care and emotional care are essential in these services and is designed in a "self-discovery" and "self delineated change" process format that is intended to empower the health providers themselves.

Contact: Maureen Chilila in Lusaka:
Tel (260) 1-253-314
Cell (260) 96-745-888

INDEX